D1564787

# Health Outcomes for Older People:
# Questions for the Coming Decade

Committee to Develop an Agenda for
Health Outcomes Research for Elderly People

Jill C. Feasley, *Editor*

Division of Health Care Services

INSTITUTE OF MEDICINE

NATIONAL ACADEMY PRESS
Washington, D.C.  1996

**National Academy Press • 2101 Constitution Avenue, N.W. • Washington, D.C. 20418**

NOTICE: The project that is the subject of this report was approved by the Governing Board of the National Research Council, whose members are drawn from the councils of the National Academy of Sciences, the National Academy of Engineering, and the Institute of Medicine. The members of the committee responsible for the report were chosen for their special competencies and with regard for appropriate balance.

This report has been reviewed by a group other than the authors according to procedures approved by a Report Review Committee consisting of members of the National Academy of Sciences, the National Academy of Engineering, and the Institute of Medicine.

The Institute of Medicine was established in 1970 by the National Academy of Sciences to secure the services of eminent members of appropriate professions in the examination of policy matters pertaining to the health of the public. The Institute acts under the responsibility given to the National Academy of Sciences by its congressional charter to be an adviser to the federal government and, upon its own initiative, to identify issues of medical care, research, and education. Dr. Kenneth Shine is president of the Institute of Medicine.

Support for this project was provided by the Greenwall Foundation and the National Research Council. The views presented are those of the Institute of Medicine Committee to Develop an Agenda for Health Outcomes Research for Elderly People and are not necessarily those of the funding organizations.

International Standard Book No. 0-309-05636-5

Additional copies of this report are available from:

National Academy Press
2101 Constitution Avenue, N.W.
Box 285
Washington, DC 20055

Call (800) 624-6242 or (202) 334-3313 (in the Washington metropolitan area).

*Study Staff*

**Jill Feasley**, Program Officer
**Marilyn Field**, Deputy Director, Division of Health Care Services
**Chloe Brooke**, Intern
**Richard Julian**, Project Assistant
**Annice Hirt**, Administrative Assistant
**Clyde Behney**, Director, Division of Health Care Services

# Preface

The nation's press made much ado recently when President Clinton celebrated his 50th birthday. As one of the first baby boomers to become eligible for membership in the American Association of Retired Persons, the president symbolized how close the demographic bulge in the American population known as the "Baby Boom" is getting to senior citizenship.

The implications for American society as baby boomers become senior citizens in the coming decades are sizable. The rising cost of medical care in this country is already on a collision course with both the Medicare trust fund and the public's desire to limit taxes, even before the first boomers have reached Medicare eligibility. Modern medicine's capacity to avert death from acute diseases converts these diseases into chronic conditions that will, in turn, command even more of the health care budget. There will be more older Americans, living longer, with more chronic diseases; and we will have more capability to treat them.

The task the Institute of Medicine assigned to the committee that developed this report was not to predict the future but rather to suggest a framework for developing new understanding of the outcomes of health care for older people. We will increasingly face a bewildering number of choices—ranging from which type of health plan to join to what type of care to follow when we are ill or dying. It is this committee's hope that as we choose among these options we can do so with solid information about the likely results or outcomes of our decisions.

Interest in examining health outcomes is not new. Indeed at *the beginning of this century*, a young surgeon in Boston named Ernest Amory Codman pioneered and actively advocated the use of his "end results idea," which he later described as

> the common-sense notion that every hospital should follow *every* patient it treats, long enough to determine whether or not the treatment has been successful. And then to inquire "if not, why not" with a view to preventing similar failures in the future.[*]

Over the decades, this common-sense notion has guided important advances in the conduct of health outcomes research. Today's researchers can determine much more than simply whether a patient lived or died after receiving a particular treatment. With a continuously growing assortment of measurement instruments and tools at their disposal, they can examine a treatment's effect on a person's overall quality of life and ability to function—physically, cognitively, and socially. Research funded by both the public and the private sector has produced ways of carrying out sophisticated quantitative and qualitative analysis, and sources of information about health are increasingly being stored in large computerized databases.

The results of health outcomes research have wide applicability. Individuals and their families can base important decisions about treatment goals on information about the health outcomes of patients with similar conditions. Practitioners can use models developed by health outcomes researchers to predict a patient's future level of functioning and to select appropriate interventions. Administrators of health plans and integrated delivery systems can study ways to reduce costs while improving the quality of care delivery. Policymakers can devise reimbursement incentives to help achieve desired outcomes.

Yet, many questions remain unanswered or unexplored. These questions form the basis of the agenda of research topics presented in this report. The committee believes these topics warrant attention from the policy and research communities—and from the public- and private-sector funders of research—within the next few years. Although older people are the focus of this agenda, the research endorsed here will benefit young and old alike if it succeeds in advancing the field of health outcomes research and in improving the way health

---

[*] E.A. Codman, *The Shoulder: Rupture of the Supraspinatus Tendon and Other Lesions in or about the Subacromial Bursa* (Boston: Thomas Todd Company, 1934), cited in L.I. Iezzoni, *Risk Adjustment for Measuring Health Care Outcomes* (Ann Arbor, Mich.: Health Administration Press, 1994).

care is provided. The report is offered in the hope that an effective outcomes research strategy will maximize the returns from the nation's health care enterprise and its biomedical research investment.

John M. Eisenberg, M.D., *Chair*
*Committee to Develop an Agenda for*
*Health Outcomes Research for Elderly People*

# Acknowledgments

Special thanks are due to several individuals to whom the committee and staff are particularly indebted. Kathleen Lohr, former director of the Institute of Medicine's (IOM) Division of Health Care Services and current senior director of Health Services Research at the Research Triangle Institute, oversaw the initial work on this project and continued to provide helpful and timely advice even after she assumed her current duties. Holly Dawkins, former research assistant, also provided support at the project's beginning before relocating to South Carolina. They are both greatly missed by their colleagues.

Initial direction for this study was provided by a planning group that met in April 1996. That meeting was chaired by Roger Herdman, IOM senior scholar, and the participants were Elena Andresen, Molla Donaldson, Pamela Doty, Charles J. Fahey, Marilyn Field, Anne Jackson, Stephen F. Jencks, Claire Macklan, Vincent Mor, Connie Pechura, Linda Redford, Paul Schyve, Cathy Sherbourne, Albert Siu, William Stubing, Eric Tangalos, Joan Teno, Jürgen Unützer, and William Weissert. Meeting participants ate lunch with a group of senior citizens attending the IONA Senior Services/St. Mary's Court lunch program in the Foggy Bottom neighborhood of Washington, D.C. Lillian Gordon, the program's site manager, graciously hosted our crowd with her renowned aplomb and style. We are especially thankful to the older people who spoke with us after lunch for their willingness to discuss the health care issues they felt would be most important to address over the next decade.

# Contents

# Summary

## OVERVIEW

In the future, how will older Americans and their families make decisions about important health care choices? Early in 1996, the Greenwall Foundation asked the Institute of Medicine (IOM) to propose an agenda for health outcomes research focused on older people to provide the information to make those decisions. This report contains the response to that request as devised by a 17-member IOM committee. It considers what the future is likely to bring for America's older population, its health care system, and the field of health outcomes research; and it presents the committee's recommendations for research to be undertaken over the next 10 years. As used in this report, **health outcomes research is research that studies the end results of the structure and processes of health care on the health and well-being of patients and populations.**

Older individuals and their families enter the health care system with their own unique set of problems, conditions, and values. Like younger people, however, they vary in their circumstances and their preferences for different outcomes; these variations need to be considered both in providing health care and in evaluating its effects on the health and well-being of older people. A basic challenge of health outcomes research is discovering how to draw general conclusions about health care and health outcomes that are still sensitive to differences in what people need and desire from the health care system. If the recommendations contained in this agenda are realized, the field of health outcomes research will be better prepared with the measurement tools and information needed to meet that challenge and to identify positive and negative conse-

1

quences of the major changes now under way in health care delivery and financing in the United States.

The committee identified two types of *outcomes measures* for special research attention over the next 10 years. They are: (1) *health-related quality of life, including functional health status,*72) *satisfaction with care.* For most older individuals, health-related quality of life—with its focus on an individual's perceptions and judgments about his or her life—is perhaps the most important outcome to consider.

Central to all research examining health outcomes are reliable, valid, and practical measurement tools. The committee recommends the development of a "toolbox" of well-defined and validated measurement instruments that have been specifically tested for use with older individuals in different care settings, including nursing homes. In one of its most significant recommendations, the committee calls for the development of a core set of outcomes indicators for practitioners, health care plans, and organizations to use in monitoring health outcomes for the older individuals and populations they serve. It also recommends further research on how outcomes data can be made more clinically relevant and useful in correcting deficiencies in processes or systems of care.

Development of such a core set of indicators will involve investigation of practice variations, patient and consumer involvement in care decisionmaking, and strategies for disseminating outcomes information and changing practice patterns. It will also require attention to the impact of changes in the current systems of financing, service delivery, and quality assessment and improvement. The committee recommended that research focus in particular on changes in health outcomes that may occur as older individuals make transitions, such as when they move between types of care (e.g., from active treatment to palliative care), treatment settings, and health plans.

In order to improve the scope and quality of health outcomes research, several basic infrastructure issues also need to be addressed. In particular, tackling the research questions posed in this report calls for a well-trained research workforce, continued work to improve research strategies and measurement tools, and efforts to preserve and improve the integrity of research and the quality of outcomes data.

The complete list of the committee's recommendations follows.

## RECOMMENDATIONS: RESEARCH ISSUES

### Health-Related Quality of Life

*Health-related quality of life should be a major focus of health outcomes research for older individuals. The research should continue to examine how to define and measure those dimensions of health-related quality of life that are particularly important to older individuals. In particular, more and better global and targeted functional measures should be developed for older individuals to describe and assess functional outcomes (a) in general, (b) for distinct clinical conditions, and (c) within specific settings.*

### Satisfaction with Care

*Improvements should be made in the way older individuals' satisfaction with care is measured and interpreted.*

### "Toolbox" of Outcomes Measures and a Core Set of Outcomes Measures

*A well-defined set or "toolbox" of outcomes measures for older individuals should be developed and further refined. The toolbox should allow easy and appropriate application of these measurement tools by nonresearchers in a variety of settings. A core set of outcomes measures should be developed for use by practitioners, health care plans, and organizations serving older individuals and populations. Methods of making outcomes data more useful clinically should be developed.*

### Practice Patterns and Interventions and Their Effect on Outcomes

*Continued research should examine how different practice patterns and treatment interventions affect older individuals' health outcomes. Specific examples of practice patterns and interventions to study include advance care planning; clinical practice guidelines, pathways, and other strategies; and interdisciplinary intervention teams. An examination of the cost-effectiveness of these practices should be included.*

### Involvement in Care Decisionmaking

*Methods of enhancing older individuals' and their families' involvement in decisionmaking about their care and its relationship to health outcomes should be tested.*

## Education and Dissemination of Outcomes Information

*The effectiveness and impact on health outcomes of providing health care information to older individuals and health care professionals should be evaluated. New and improved ways of disseminating outcomes information should be tested.*

## Financing Systems

*Research, including randomized controlled trials and quasi-experiments, should continue to examine how various provider payment methods and programs affect the health outcomes of older individuals and populations. Outcomes of special concern are access to care, health care costs, quality of care, health-related quality of life, functional health status, and satisfaction with care.*

## Service Delivery and Utilization

*As alternative forms of organizing and delivering health care for older individuals are encouraged and continue to be developed, the effect on health outcomes should receive continuing and rigorous evaluation.*

## Transitions

*The impact on health outcomes when older individuals make transitions between types of care (e.g., from active treatment to palliative care), treatment settings, and health plans should be explored.*

## Quality Assessment and Improvement

*The performance of the government regulatory agencies, private-sector accreditation organizations, and organizations' internal programs in using outcomes-based quality assessment and improvement systems should be evaluated for effectiveness in improving health outcomes for older populations.*

## RECOMMENDATIONS: RESEARCH INFRASTRUCTURE NEEDS

### Workforce Issues

*Government agencies and private foundations should support training and education opportunities in health outcomes research.*

## Conduct of Research

*Principles for the appropriate conduct of health outcomes research and the use and dissemination of outcomes data need to be developed and implemented.*

## Data Quality

*Research on the quality of data used in health outcomes research should be supported.*

## Data Management Systems

*An independent appraisal of systems for data management that support outcomes research should be conducted. This includes evaluations of specific tools and applications, informatics, databases, and basic telecommunications infrastructure.*

## Methodological and Analytic Issues

*Continued support should be provided to develop advances in the methodology and analysis used in health outcomes research.*

Viewpoint remains that of health professionals "managing" patients, occasionally letting them participate in decision-making. Need to get outside this closed perspective and recognize how much of the process is self-initiated and -directed.

# Introduction and Background

## HEALTH OUTCOMES RESEARCH
## FOR OLDER PEOPLE

A key question to answer in the coming decade is "How can the unique needs and desires of each person be appropriately assessed and addressed in a rapidly changing health care environment?" Health outcomes research has the potential of providing the measurement tools to make that assessment and the analytic knowledge to suggest ways of addressing the challenges posed.

This report presents an agenda of health outcomes research for older people, proposed to be undertaken over the next 10 years. As used in this report, **health outcomes research is research that studies the end results of the structure and processes of health care on the health and well-being of patients and populations.** Its objectives are to provide information and insights to guide health care improvements, promote efficiency, and reduce costs. The research itself can be conducted on many different levels, ranging from that of an individual's health status to that of the broadly defined health care system, and usually employs a multidisciplinary approach.

The term "outcomes" has come into wide use in a variety of contexts. Health outcomes can also be represented by specific measures, including those that focus on:

- clinical signs or symptoms (physiologic and biologic);
- well-being or mental and emotional functioning;
- physical, cognitive, and social functioning;
- satisfaction with care;

- health-related quality of life; and
- costs and appropriate use of resources.

Beyond these basic terms and concepts, the formulation of an outcomes research agenda requires a consideration of what the future is likely to bring for America's older population, its health care system, and the field of health outcomes research.

### An Expanding Older Population

America's demographic future is relatively easy to predict. On May 19, 2011, "baby boomers" start turning 65 (*Time*, 1986). In that year, those over age 65 will constitute nearly 14 percent of the U.S. population and are projected to increase to over 20 percent by the year 2030 (U.S. Bureau of the Census, 1996). In contrast, today 12.8 percent of the population are in this age group. The aging boomers, now in their middle age, will continue to have a significant impact on American society and to challenge the health care delivery and financing systems.

On the furthest end of the aging spectrum, the demographic impact of an aging population is even more striking. The oldest of the old, people 85 years old and over, are the fastest growing segment of the older population. Those over the age of 85 currently make up 1.4 percent of the population, a figure that will increase to 2.4 percent by the year 2030. This is significant because this segment typically has the most health impairments and highest per capita health costs. Women are likely to remain disproportionately represented in older age groups, especially the oldest of the old. Today women make up nearly 60 percent of the elderly population and account for more than 70 percent of the oldest of the old. Although the ratio of elderly men to women is expected to narrow slowly over the coming decades, in the year 2030 women will still account for more than 54 percent of the elderly population and more than 64 percent of those age 85 and older.

The older population is, moreover, projected to be much more racially and ethnically diverse than ever before. The current elderly population is predominantly white. However, demographers project that by the middle of the next century the numbers of elderly blacks will more than triple, increasing their proportion of the total elderly population from 8 to 10 percent. And more dramatically, the Hispanic population will increase nearly 11-fold, rising from less than 4 percent of the elderly to nearly 16 percent. The projected increases in minority population will cause the proportion of white elderly to shrink from more than 86 percent to less than 67 percent.

While many older people lead robust and active lives in relatively good health, some general characteristics tend to differentiate them from younger people. These factors include a greater likelihood of having multiple clinical conditions (and subsequent use of multiple medications) and a variety of sensory, mobility, and cognitive impairments (e.g., poor vision or hearing, gait instability). Health outcomes related to quality-of-life issues become more striking as one ages, particularly as older people and their families confront issues about dying and care at the end of life. Many older people live alone, which, when overlaid with poor health, increases their sense of vulnerability and raises concerns about their ability to get needed support for tasks ranging from going to medical appointments to preparing food to having someone to discuss their preferences about care. Again, these are general characteristics. The older population, with an age range spanning more than 30 years, is quite diverse and heterogeneous.

## Changing Health Care Environment

To assert that today's health care environment is dynamic is to risk understatement. The pressure to contain costs and add value to health care spending has led to new ways of paying health care providers and practitioners, new ways of managing patient access to health care providers, and new ways of delivering services. Significant restructuring is being proposed for the Medicare and Medicaid programs, which finance considerable portions of the health care costs for older Americans. For example, the incentives for Medicare beneficiaries to join managed care plans are likely to become stronger and may, depending on their specific characteristics, dramatically restructure the current Medicare program. Many state Medicaid programs have already moved in this direction.

Hospitals, nursing facilities, home health agencies, and health maintenance organizations are preparing to meet the demands of the changing size and composition of the older population in an environment likely to be characterized by major resource constraints. Policymakers continue to examine ways to ensure quality and accessibility of care in such an environment (IOM, 1990, 1994; WHCOA, 1996). How the growing older population interacts with the health care system is also changing. More than ever before, the attitudes of older people and their families about outcomes of health care and the processes used to achieve them are being identified and taken into account. The demographic trends described above are likely to contribute to critical change in practices and expectations about health care.

## Field of Health Outcomes Research

The field of health outcomes research itself is also dynamic. In the past two decades, and especially in the past five years, major advances have been made—

particularly in assessing functional health status and quality-of-life outcomes. The progress has come principally on two fronts:

1. an increased understanding of the need to measure a full range of health states, using information directly from individuals (or their proxies) so that the effects of health care and health care policy can be more fully and accurately discerned; and
2. an expanded inventory of measurement tools, including an array of reliable, valid, and practical questionnaires and other instruments to assess health outcomes that are meaningful to people in their daily lives.

The results of health outcomes research are used in many ways. Individuals can use them to help make their own decisions about which course of treatment to follow or which health plan to join. Practitioners can use models developed by health outcomes researchers to predict a patient's future level of functioning and to select appropriate interventions. Administrators of health plans and integrated delivery systems can study ways to reduce costs while improving the quality of care delivery. Policymakers can devise reimbursement incentives to help achieve desired outcomes.

Health outcomes research is not without its critics. For example, some question certain uses of quality-of-life measures out of concern that they may denigrate those with disabilities. Others express concerns about manipulation of patient satisfaction measures, neglect of process-of-care measures, and inattention to aspects of health for which data are not readily available. Brook et al. (1996) argue that process measures are more sensitive measures of quality of care because poor outcomes may not occur each time something is done incorrectly or something is omitted that should have been done, such as giving thrombolytic therapy to appropriate myocardial patients. In addition, outcomes often take a long time to occur and can require very large samples to measure a statistically significant effect.

Health outcomes research is funded both publicly and privately. Within the federal government, the Agency for Health Care Policy and Research (AHCPR) has been designated the lead agency with responsibility for funding health outcomes research. Under AHCPR's stewardship, major advances in the field of health outcomes research have been supported and the results widely disseminated. Despite recent significant budget cutbacks, AHCPR continues to fund several Patient Outcomes Research Teams (PORTs) through its Medical Treatment Effectiveness Program. PORTs allow multidisciplinary teams of researchers to focus their combined expertise on the outcomes and costs of alternative practice patterns in treating a particular health condition.

Elsewhere in the federal government, health outcomes research is being funded by a variety of agencies and departments, including the Health Care Financing Administration, the National Institutes of Health, the Health Resources and Services Administration, and the Department of Veterans Affairs. It is difficult to identify the amount of overall federal research dollars devoted specifically to health outcomes for older individuals. In general, federal funding for health *services* research (of which health outcomes research can be considered a part) is much lower than for federal biomedical research; in fiscal year 1994, federal health services research received $470 million in support compared to $10 billion for federal biomedical research. Certainly some biomedical research can be considered health outcomes research, but it often only examines traditional outcomes such as mortality and typically does not take into account the more sophisticated measures of health status and functional outcomes that are particularly important in the older population. Additionally, older people are often deliberately excluded from this type of clinical research.

Some state and local governments also support health outcomes research, most notably California, New York, and Pennsylvania. Likewise, private foundations, including the Commonwealth, Greenwall, John A. Hartford, Henry J. Kaiser Family, Pew Charitable Trusts, and Robert Wood Johnson foundations, have supported important research examining health outcomes for older individuals. Finally, private health care organizations—large and small—continue to support certain kinds of health outcomes research to analyze and improve health care for older people and their families.

## ORIGINS OF THIS REPORT AND STUDY APPROACH

A rich set of research questions emerges from the combination of the important policy questions introduced above. Early in 1996, the Greenwall Foundation approached the Institute of Medicine (IOM) about the possibility of convening an expert committee to examine these questions and to propose an agenda for health outcomes research focused on older people. The Greenwall Foundation, founded in 1949 and based in New York City, typically funds medical research in bone cancer, diabetes, and geriatrics. It also funds studies of bioethics and the moral dilemmas involved in medical decisionmaking, which led to its current interest in health outcomes research. Rather than fund individual health outcomes research projects, officials of the Greenwall Foundation felt it would be more beneficial to promote and help fund projects that were part of a coherent and comprehensive strategy of research designed to truly advance the field of health outcomes research. The IOM committee that developed this agenda understood that it would be the basis for discussions with other foundations and agencies and for efforts to leverage funds to achieve the greatest benefit on the health outcomes of older people.

Preliminary ideas for the committee's work and workshop were formulated during a special planning meeting sponsored by the IOM in April 1996. After that meeting, the IOM appointed a 17-member committee to oversee the entire process. The committee included individuals with expertise in geriatrics and

12 HEALTH OUTCOMES FOR OLDER PEOPLE

gerontology, nursing, social work, dentistry, epidemiology, consumer and patient advocacy, health care financing and delivery, and health outcomes research (see page iii). The committee sponsored a one-day invitational workshop in Washington, D.C. (see Appendix for the workshop agenda and participants list) and met the following day to discuss the information presented and develop their recommendations. The committee then reviewed and commented on successive drafts of the final report.

Several processes informed the committee's work. These involved a thorough review of the relevant literature; presentations given at the invitational workshop that included input from consumers, leading researchers, and government officials; commissioned papers; and the actual deliberations of the committee and the discussion of members' expert opinions. These processes helped to identify 10 recommendations for research issues and 5 recommendations for research infrastructure needs.

In evaluating their recommendations, the committee considered the potential of the ensuing research to:

- improve individuals' health outcomes,
- affect a large population,
- address important social or ethical questions,
- affect policy decisions,
- enhance the national capacity for health outcomes research, or
- be readily conducted.

The committee recognizes that the cost of care is an outcome of considerable importance. Clinicians routinely include costs in their consideration of outcomes when recommending alternative therapies to older patients and families. Government and private payers are acutely focused on issues of cost because failure to use resources wisely will ultimately reduce the availability of care, access to care, and the effectiveness of care. For those reasons, the committee recommends that all outcomes research attempt to determine the costs associated with the outcomes achieved. This information will help patients, practitioners, and policymakers to make more informed decisions about the trade-offs involved in achieving desired outcomes. In a similar vein, the committee does not specifically single out the need for research on more traditional mortality and preventable morbidity measures. These measures have been and continue to be important; they also have been and continue to be the subject of much research. The committee decided, therefore, to highlight areas that have received less attention.

The committee considered several other research agendas on aging issues that have been developed by other groups. A 1991 IOM publication, *Extending Life, Enhancing Life: A National Research Agenda on Aging*, presented a 20-year agenda of age-related research. In 1995, the federal Task Force on Aging

Research released *Threshold of Discovery*, a prioritized agenda of some 192 research recommendations for the federal government to undertake within the next five years. Both of these research agendas broadly covered all aspects of aging from basic biomedical research to assistive technology development to studies of transportation needs. As such, neither focused specifically on health outcomes research per se. Nonetheless, these agendas have been useful in heightening awareness of research needs in the entire field of aging and in building consensus about research priorities. Indeed, substantial progress has been made in carrying out some of the research recommended, and new priorities have surfaced.

## AUDIENCE FOR THIS REPORT

Implementation of the recommendations for research contained in this report will require the combined efforts of many individuals and organizations. Funding will need to come from federal, state, and local governments, private industry, and foundations. Therefore, the research recommendations contained in this report are aimed at a variety of very different potential funders. The committee recognized that no single funder would be likely to support all the research identified here; each funder will have different priorities and research interests. The research itself will need to be conducted by health outcomes researchers working in a variety of health care organizations, universities, government agencies, and private-sector accreditation organizations—sometimes working independently, sometimes working collaboratively.

## ORGANIZATION OF THIS REPORT

An "agenda" can be defined as "a list of things to be done," and it is in this sense of the word that the current work is presented. Final recommendations have been organized into two main categories: research issues and research infrastructure needs. All recommendations selected for this report have been deemed to be of a high priority to pursue over the next 10 years; the committee did not rank order the recommendations. Thus, the order in which they are presented here does not imply any priorities among them. Naturally, some overlap exists among the various recommendations, and the committee has acknowledged interrelations at several points.

Each recommendation is listed individually in the following standard format:

- Recommendation,
- Rationale,
- Background, and
- Examples of Needed Research.

A bibliography, which appears at the end of the report, provides selected references pertinent to each recommendation. These references supplement those cited in the text, and they are listed at the end of each chapter. Their inclusion is intended to guide readers to a few key resources on particular areas. Again, the reference list in the bibliography is not meant to provide an exhaustive review.

## REFERENCES

Brook, R.H., C.J. Kamberg, and E.A. McGlynn. Health System Reform and Quality. *Journal of the American Medical Association* 276(6):476–480, 1996.

IOM (Institute of Medicine). *Medicare: A Strategy for Quality Assurance.* K. Lohr, ed. Washington, D.C.: National Academy Press, 1990.

IOM. *Extending Life, Enhancing Life: A National Research Agenda on Aging.* E.T. Lonergan, ed. Washington, D.C.: National Academy Press, 1991.

IOM. *Access to Health Care in America.* M. Millman, ed. Washington, D.C.: National Academy Press, 1994.

Task Force on Aging Research. *The Threshold of Discovery: Future Directions for Research on Aging.* Administrative Document. Report of the Task Force on Aging Research. Washington, D.C.: Department of Health and Human Services, April 1995.

*Time*, The Baby Boomers Turn 40. May 19, 1986.

U.S. Bureau of the Census. Current Population Reports, Series P25-1130. *Population Projections of the United States by Age, Sex, Race, and Hispanic Origin: 1995 to 2050.* Washington, D.C.: U.S. Government Printing Office, 1996.

White House Conference on Aging (WHCOA). *The Road to an Aging Policy for the 21st Century: Final Report of the 1995 White House Conference on Aging.* Washington, D.C.: WHCOA, 1996.

# Recommendations:
# Research Issues

Older individuals and their families enter the health care system with their own unique set of problems and conditions. How well these characteristics are addressed significantly influences the individuals' ultimate health outcomes. In the research world, these intrinsic and extrinsic characteristics can be thought of as independent variables. In the day-to-day world of older individuals and their families, they can be thought of as the circumstances in which people find themselves. A basic challenge of health outcomes research is discovering how to draw generalized conclusions about the relationship of causes (e.g., treatments, policy decisions) and effects or outcomes while recognizing that each person's circumstances are unique and that some variation is to be expected. People have different preferences for different outcomes, and those differences need to be identified and, whenever possible, honored.

To support those efforts, the committee recommends that the following 10 areas receive concentrated attention over the next 10 years:

- **Health-Related Quality of Life**
- **Satisfaction with Care**
- **"Toolbox" of Outcomes Measures and a Core Set of Outcomes Measures**
- **Practice Patterns and Interventions and Their Effect on Outcomes**
- **Involvement in Care Decisionmaking**
- **Education and Dissemination of Outcomes Information**
- **Financing Systems**
- **Service Delivery and Utilization**
- **Transitions**
- **Quality Assessment and Improvement**

## HEALTH-RELATED QUALITY OF LIFE

*Health-related quality of life should be a major focus of health out-*
*comes research for older individuals. This research should continue*
*to examine how to define and measure those dimensions of health-*
*related quality of life that are particularly important to older indi-*
*viduals. In particular, more and better global and targeted functional*
*measures should be developed for older individuals to describe and*
*assess functional outcomes (a) in general, (b) for distinct clinical*
*conditions, and (c) within specific settings.*

### Rationale

• Health-related quality of life is perhaps the most important dimension of health outcomes for older individuals. Traditionally, the goal of health care has been to treat acute illness and delay or avert death. Increasingly, however, the goal of many older individuals and their families is not simply to add "years to life" but also to add "life to years."

• Although the importance of assessing health-related quality of life for older individuals is increasingly being recognized, it remains a difficult concept to measure validly or reliably, especially among the older segments of these populations and for those with cognitive or communicative impairments.

• Several instruments have been developed to measure health-related quality of life, but more needs to be known about how accurately they take into account older peoples' values, perceptions, and preferences and how contextual factors affect measurements.

• Functional health status is a significant dimension of health-related quality of life for older individuals. Maintenance of function or the slowing of deterioration in function may be the primary goal of treatment of many older people, especially those with multiple health conditions.

• Targeted measures are needed to compare the efficacy and effectiveness of new interventions and to assess the impact of particular diseases and impairments (e.g., measuring the ability of arthritis patients' to walk without pain or the ability of patients with dental disease to chew food). The relative importance of certain aspects of functional status varies by setting; indeed, functional status is a key factor determining a person's setting (e.g., where not having adequate cognitive functioning to live independently in the community requires residing in an institution).

### Background

For the vast majority of older individuals, quality of life may have nothing to do with health care delivery. However, many quality-of-life issues do relate to health care and many health outcomes are influenced by an individual's overall quality of life. This committee has chosen to define health-related quality of life as "a personal perception characterizing the way an individual feels about his or her health status, including physical, psychological, religious, and social domains of health status." This definition incorporates or overlaps with several other types of outcomes, including functional health status and satisfaction with care. It is also meant to capture the effect of a variety of other perceptions, including autonomy, vitality, vulnerability, well-being, and sense of isolation or marginalization.

Contextual factors have an effect on health-related quality of life. These refer to an older individual's environment and include a constellation of factors such as the availability of and access to appropriate health care, transportation, caregiving arrangements, culture, and social and community support. They also refer to the type of setting an individual is in, whether it be a hospital, nursing facility, assisted living facility, or single-family home. The relative importance of the various dimensions of health-related quality of life often differ depending on the context or setting. For example, among older persons in nursing homes, health-related quality of life may include the ability to make decisions, have control over their daily schedule, and maintain a sense of dignity and privacy.

Although few people question the importance of quality of life, most researchers outside the field of health outcomes research still find this a rather abstract and subjective concept. Despite the increase in the use of the term "health-related quality of life" and a proliferation of measures that attempt to capture this domain, no theoretical framework fully explains why and how disease and disability influence quality of life. Most articles addressing quality of life give only brief or superficial definitions of the construct, if any at all.

Finally, assessment of health-related quality of life needs to be based on the values and preferences of older individuals. Some widely used instruments, such as the Quality of Well-Being Scale, rate death as the worst functional outcome. Patrick and colleagues (1994) point out, however, that many patients believe there are some health states worse than death, such as being in a persistive vegetative state. In those cases, death—especially death with dignity—might actually be the individual's preferred health status outcome. Some instruments, such as the Health Utility Index, do incorporate health states worse than death and are beginning to be more widely used.

*Functional Health Status*

Functional health status is an important dimension of health-related quality of life. It refers to an individual's ability to perform certain types of activities.

Assessing functional health status involves an evaluation of three areas:

1. physical functioning,
2. psychological functioning (including cognitive functioning, mental health, coping ability, and sense of autonomy), and
3. social functioning.

As individuals age, their likelihood of developing a pathology, that is, a specific disease, that interrupts or interferes with normal bodily processes or structures increases. Indeed, the older a person becomes the more likely he or she is to develop several such conditions (often referred to as comorbidities), particularly ones that are chronic or long lasting. Additionally, as an individual ages he or she is more likely to experience sensory and other impairments, such as poor vision or hearing. These diseases or impairments can lead to functional limitations that restrict an individual's ability to perform an action or activity in the manner or within the range that is considered normal. The cumulative effect of this process results in disability: the inability or limitation in performing socially defined activities and roles expected of individuals within a social and physical environment (IOM, 1991). The following conceptualization depicts this process. Although it is not depicted here, the environment also plays a key role in determining the severity of this disabling process.

Pathology → Impairment → Functional Limitation → Disability

A great deal of medical research has examined how the first two components of this conceptualization—pathology and impairment—affect older individuals' health outcomes. The committee believes this research is vital and ultimately should be conducted for all the diseases and impairments that commonly affect older individuals. The committee did not, however, attempt to prioritize which specific clinical conditions should be examined within the next 10 years. Such prioritization has been done before, however. Although not specifically focused on aging issues, the Institute of Medicine developed a model process for picking clinical conditions and technologies to be given priority research funding in a series of reports on effectiveness research (IOM, 1989, 1990a,b,d). Additionally, the federal Task Force on Aging Research (1995) recently released a comprehensive agenda for aging research, including a prioritized listing of research needed on specific diseases, disabilities, and mental disorders (albeit not necessarily with a focus on outcomes).

In general, the committee supports the type of basic biomedical research called for in those reports, with the caveat that older individuals need to be included in related clinical trials. Older people are often deliberately excluded from clinical research. Even when older individuals are included in clinical trials, interpreting the findings can be difficult. Variability in outcomes may be inadequately explained even after age differences within the older population are taken into account.

Often as individuals age, however, understanding a particular disease or impairment becomes less important than understanding how it affects an individual's ability to function, as portrayed in the last two components of the above conceptualization—functional limitation and disability. Naturally, the severity and limitation or burden imposed by these diseases and impairments varies by individual and, in part, determines the extent to which the diseases or impairment become a disability. It is also important to understand the relative contribution to the effect of each individual disease or impairment on function.

The committee considers a focus on overall functional outcomes essential to the everyday work of practitioners and care providers when assessing the merits of medical interventions and quality of medical care for older individuals. Yet, important measurement issues exist. For example, most current measurement tools are used to assess a patient's functioning at a single point in time; the focus needs to be redirected to how functioning changes over time. These concerns must be addressed before practitioners can begin widespread use of these measurement and assessment tools.

### Examples of Needed Research

- Construct a better theoretical model of the dimensions of health-related quality of life most important to older persons, include a consideration of how these dimensions might change in different settings.
- Develop a compendium of health-related quality-of-life measurement instruments specifically for older people (see also the recommendation on a "toolbox" of outcomes measures).
- Support more longitudinal research on older individuals' health-related quality of life.
- Investigate the major predictors of functional decline or improvement and the relationship between functional limitation and disability.
- Conduct longitudinal research on function change over time.
- Develop models to better predict future functioning.
- Analyze how functional health outcomes are affected when an individual has multiple diseases and impairments.
- Examine how current and new measures of functional health status help differentiate health care plans and practitioners.
- Compile measures of functional health status and evaluate their appropriateness for use with older individuals.

## SATISFACTION WITH CARE

*Improvements should be made in the way older individuals' satisfaction with care is measured and interpreted.*

### Rationale

• Satisfaction with care is a significant dimension of health-related quality of life for older individuals.

• Satisfaction is increasingly being measured as a way to judge quality—and determine payment—for both individual practitioners and health plans.

• The relationship between satisfaction with care and other outcomes of interest is not well known.

• Despite progress, available measurement tools and analytic methods of interpreting satisfaction with care can lead to spurious interpretations and conclusions.

### Background

*Measuring Satisfaction*

Several instruments already exist to measure overall *ratings* of care (i.e., asking patients to rate their care as either "poor to excellent" or to say whether they are "very dissatisfied" or "very satisfied"). These instruments are widely used throughout the health care industry. However, a variety of methodological issues need to be addressed. These include issues of question phrasing, item placement, appropriate response choices, and whether the care being rated is the last visit versus all visits in the past year. The satisfaction scores from some instruments are often skewed toward the "very good" to "excellent" responses; this has been shown to be particularly true when older individuals are surveyed. Yet the real difference between rating care as "very good" rather than "excellent" might be underestimated. Getting a "very good" response may be an early warning sign of problems and provide an opportunity for further examination into ways to improve care. Moreover, lack of a clear understanding of these distinctions makes it difficult to establish a credible benchmark of satisfaction against which to measure improvement.

Some cognitive research of survey respondents is already being undertaken to understand better the process by which patients respond to questions about the rating of medical care.[1] Such research is important. It is equally important

---

[1] For example, this type of research is being undertaken as part of a recently funded study of consumer assessments of health plans. The Agency for Health Care Policy and Research is the sponsoring agency, and the study is being conducted by a consortium of researchers from Harvard University, the RAND Corporation, and the Research Triangle Institute.

that conceptual models of the cognitive process used in determining whether one is satisfied be expanded or further developed. To date, researchers have drawn on job satisfaction and marketing research models to develop similar models in health care.

In terms of *reports* of specific care events, further refinement and use of patient surveys to capture actual health experiences, not just "satisfaction" with the experiences, is needed. The Picker-Commonwealth Foundation (Cleary et al., 1991) developed a 61-item survey about patients' experience of hospital care that was based solely on patient reports of specific events (e.g., "Were you told of the purpose of your medications in a way that you could understand?"). This survey, which examines hospital care from the perspectives of seven domains (including respect for patients' values, preferences, and expressed needs; coordination and integration of care; physical comfort; transitions; and continuity of care) was developed based on focus groups and expert panel review. Use of such reports minimizes the influence of confounding factors such as patients' expectations, personal relationships, practitioners' style, gratitude, or response tendencies related to gender, class, or ethnicity.

The committee believes it is important to measure both patients' overall *ratings* of satisfaction and their *reports* of care events to understand more accurately the factors that influence an individual's sense of satisfaction. For example, a patient and his or her family could report quite factually that a physician discussed whether life-sustaining treatment should be utilized. Yet, their rating of satisfaction with that conversation may be quite different depending on the physician's skill and sensitivity.

*Interpreting Satisfaction*

Interpreting the results of satisfaction surveys will involve gaining a keener understanding of patients' characteristics and their expectations of care. For example, Greenfield and colleagues (1996) examined the patient satisfaction scores of a large sample of diabetic patients. Although the scores were uniformly rather high, further analysis showed that a significant amount of the variance between scores could be attributed to the passivity of the patients and the severity of their conditions; more passive and more severely ill people were less likely to express dissatisfaction. Likewise, there appear to be generational differences in people's ratings of satisfaction. Today's 70- and 80-year-old individuals are more likely than younger people to have been socialized to avoid dissent and criticism of practitioners and the health care system. An adjustment that accounts for salient patient characteristics and illness severity seems appropriate.

Similarly, Desbiens et al. (forthcoming) noted that seriously ill patients will report both severe pain and high levels of satisfaction with their pain control. A better understanding of people's expectations might help explain this seeming incongruence. Do dying patients expect to be in pain? Would patients continue to rate their satisfaction so highly after seeing an educational video that informed them that, in the majority of situations, patients do not need to suffer severe pain while dying?

Greater sophistication in measuring and interpreting satisfaction reports and ratings holds the promise of improving the way practitioners and health plans deliver care. Until this sophistication is achieved, however, reports and rates of older people's satisfaction should be regarded cautiously.

### Examples of Needed Research

• Develop standard measures of satisfaction, specifically tested for use by older individuals, that use both reports and ratings. Satisfaction measures should include both global and disease- or setting-specific assessments.

• Establish the advantages and disadvantages inherent in the use of ratings and reports of satisfaction.

• Utilize focus groups and other qualitative methods to illuminate how patient expectations influence satisfaction. Determine how satisfaction rates might change with age and other characteristics such as cultural differences.

• Establish purposes and methods for using family reports and ratings. Explore how the perspectives of patients and family members differ in both reports and ratings of health care.

• Examine how current and new measures of satisfaction help differentiate health care plans and practitioners.

• Examine how mild to moderate cognitive impairment affects older people's responses to satisfaction surveys.

• Examine older individuals' patterns of enrollment and disenrollment in health plans and how these patterns relate to satisfaction with care.

## "TOOLBOX" OF OUTCOMES MEASURES AND
## A CORE SET OF OUTCOMES MEASURES

*A well-defined set or "toolbox" of outcomes measures for older individuals should be developed and further refined. The toolbox should allow easy and appropriate application of these measurement tools by nonresearchers in a variety of settings. A core set of outcomes measures should be developed for use by practitioners, health care plans, and organizations serving older individuals and populations. Methods of making outcomes data more useful clinically should be developed.*

### Rationale

• A variety of health outcomes measures exist, but many may not have been tested specifically for older people, particularly for those with cognitive or communicative impairments.

• Use of a core set of outcomes measures can provide the basis for making clinically relevant care planning decisions, whether by hospital, home health agency, nursing home staff, primary care practitioner, patient, or family caregiver.

• These data can facilitate the transfer of information across organizational boundaries, creating a common language of assessment, as well as facilitate communication among clinical staff from different disciplines (e.g., physician, nurse, dentist, physical therapist) located within the same organization but in different settings.

• These data can be used to characterize and monitor the performance of individual practitioners, provider organizations, and integrated networks of health care organizations.

### Background

Although significant progress has been made in objectively measuring and assessing a wide spectrum of health outcomes, more and better measurement tools and analysis are needed. Once these are developed, the committee recommends that they be assembled in a way that allows easy and appropriate application by nonresearchers in a variety of settings.

Various methodologic questions must be addressed during the development of this toolbox. These include (a) the applicability of using existing outcomes measures developed for generally healthy, younger adults for an older population; (b) the creation of instruments that will assess these health outcome domains reliably, validly, and with minimum respondent burden, among persons throughout the older age span; and (c) the availability of alternative formats (e.g., questionnaires or instruments that are self-administered by paper-based instruments or by computer-assisted or touch-screen technologies, and those that are interviewer-administered (which can be face to face or by telephone) and foreign language versions.

Furthermore, less is known than might be desirable about how to meet special methodologic problems of assessing health outcomes among certain groups of older people. For individuals who are cognitively impaired, as an example, more research is needed on how best to assess their health status and who should provide the information if the individuals are unable to do so themselves. Other groups that pose a methodologic challenge include individuals in various types of residential facilities, individuals from ethnic minorities for whom English is not a first language, and very old individuals.

## Core Set of Outcomes Measures

A great deal of data about patient outcomes is already being collected. For example, Medicare and Medicaid have claims data for almost all inpatient hospital stays. In 1991 the Minimum Data Set (MDS) and Resident Assessment Instrument (RAI) were mandated as the standard assessment system for all residents in all Medicare- and Medicaid-certified nursing facilities. A similar assessment system and instrument are being developed for assisted living or board and care facilities. Rehabilitation hospitals use the Functional Impact Measure (FIM) as their standard assessment instrument. Home health agencies are just beginning to implement the Outcome Assessment Instrument Set (OASIS) to track outcomes. Unfortunately, as people move back and forth across these settings, very little information has been shared.

Many of these diverse instruments and measurement traditions have been developed independently of one another. Except for activities of daily living (ADLs), few data elements and response categories in the nursing home MDS, the rehabilitation FIM, or the home care OASIS have identical meaning or scoring. Even when examining ADLs, wording differences can, in some circumstances, cause incomparability. Differences in time frames and indicators of intensity or frequency in most measures also make combining data from different measurement tools difficult. For example, using different severity measurement systems can result in very different assessments of risk, even when used on only one individual (Iezzoni, 1994).

A core set of measures can help to overcome these problems. The core set might contain measures that address outcomes as diverse as cost, satisfaction with care, and health-related quality of life. Certainly, more specialized or targeted information to supplement the core set of measures should and will continue to be collected. For example, in some cases investigators might want to add some measures designed specifically for a given diagnosis, such as the ability of older individuals with arthritis to walk without pain. Similarly, a hospice organization may want to ask its patients more questions about pain than would be needed for someone in an assisted living facility. In other cases, the inclusion of some information, such as asking about a family's ability to care for the patient at home for some permanent residents of nursing homes, may not be needed.

Most importantly, the measures must reflect the characteristics, concerns, and preferences of older individuals. The measures should be able to be tracked over time. For example, patients with chronic obstructive pulmonary disease should be able to compare the functional health status of similar patients within and across different health plans. Additionally, appropriate guidelines need to be developed about when the responses of family members and other proxies should be used in establishing the core set of measurements. (See "Involvement in Care Decisionmaking" for examples of research needed regarding the use of proxies.)

Movement toward developing and implementing a common set of indicators is already under way. Several organizations, including JCAHO, NCQA, and the Medical Outcomes Trust, have begun to collect key indicators and measurement instruments. The technical capacity for capturing data in a variety of different ways is improving; in addition, the costs for equipment and systems as diverse as text scanning, speech recognition, and bar code reading are decreasing. Software vendors and those designing integrated information systems are focusing on portability of the clinical and financial information across traditional institutional boundaries as networks of providers develop in selected markets. All these forces bode well for the emergence of a more uniform, if not standardized, clinical data collection mechanism within and across organizations.

### Examples of Needed Research

• Develop more and better outcome measurement tools specifically tested for older people.

• Once developed, assemble a compendium of these measurement tools.

• Examine ways to ensure that data gathered from multiple sources, including proxies, are accurate.

• Develop broad consensus on which outcome measures should form the core.

• Simultaneously develop better measurement tools and analytical methods. This includes valid and reliable standard definitions, criteria, mechanisms for assessing data collection for equivalency, and data collection methods.

• Investigate ways to expand and promote the clinical and organizational utility of these measures and tools. Train providers and practitioners to collect and use health outcomes data (e.g., involve doctors in development of the core set of measures). Then determine whether having more clinically useful data actually improves data quality, reliability, and validity.

• Explore ways to minimize the data collection burden.

## PRACTICE PATTERNS AND INTERVENTIONS AND
## THEIR EFFECT ON OUTCOMES

*Continued research should examine how different practice patterns and treatment interventions affect older individuals' health outcomes. Specific examples of practice patterns and interventions to study include advance care planning; clinical practice guidelines, pathways, and other strategies; and interdisciplinary intervention teams. An examination of the cost-effectiveness of these practice patterns should be included.*

### Rationale

• Wide variations in practice patterns and procedures have been documented by region and by provider, which continue to exist even after adjusting for differences in patient characteristics.

• The relationship between these variations and health outcomes has not been adequately studied.

• The effect of organizational structure, systems, and processes on health outcomes in older individuals is often unclear.

### Background

Examining the link between specific practice patterns and health-related interventions and health status has been a traditional focus of health outcomes research. Yet even when practice patterns or interventions have been linked to good outcomes, wide variations in their use has been documented. Research documenting and explaining these variations needs to continue. The emphasis should be on producing "real-time science" that can be used immediately and can support the management tools of continuous quality improvement. Processes of care, not just individual procedures, need to be examined. The characteristics, commitment, and approach of each clinical provider of services (and each administrative person as well) are also important process variables affecting outcomes. The committee has chosen three specific examples to receive specific attention because of their importance to older people; descriptions of these examples follow.

### *Advance Care Planning*

Advance care planning allows people to become more involved in care decisionmaking and lets practitioners know their treatment preferences. Problems in increasing its use exist, however (IOM, 1994). As an example, the Study to Understand Prognoses and Preferences for Outcomes and Risks of Treatments (SUPPORT) has recently documented significant problems with care at the end of life (SUPPORT, 1995). Only 41 percent of the seriously ill patients in the study reported talking to their physicians about their prognosis or the use of cardiopulmonary resuscitation (CPR). Even when such conversations took place through standardized interviews, physicians often misunderstood patients' preferences or did not issue a do-not-resuscitate order even after patients stated a preference for one. This poor communication was associated with increased poor outcomes such as severe pain, long stays in intensive care units, and use of mechanical ventilation.

## Clinical Practice Guidelines, Pathways, and Other Strategies

In recent years, a great deal of effort has gone into identifying how best to care for patients with particular types of disabling conditions. These efforts have resulted in the development and promotion of numerous clinical practice guidelines, extended care pathways, and disease management programs. Clinical practice guidelines are "systematically developed statements to assist practitioner and patient decisions about appropriate health care for specific clinical circumstances" (IOM, 1990c, p. 8). Risk identification and disease management are population-based approaches that allow health care providers and practitioners to identify people at risk for poor outcomes and to intervene with specific programs of care (which may or may not be based on clinical practice guidelines). Extended care pathways are sets of policies and procedures that practitioners and providers use to address a disabling chronic condition over time and across settings.

Many guidelines and similar tools are not age specific; others may explicitly state that they do not apply to individuals above a certain age. These provisions are, in part, an outgrowth of the limited use of older individuals in clinical trials and the application of other criteria that exclude those with multiple health problems. Thus, the evidence base may not indicate whether or how specific guidelines or disease management programs may apply to older patients, especially those with multiple health problems.

Even when guidance is specific and relevant, simply providing practitioners with information and advice does not necessarily lead to changes in their practice (Greco and Eisenberg, 1993). Several approaches for practice change have been identified (e.g., role models, feedback of information on practice patterns, changes in provider payment) that would appear to be generally relevant for those caring for older people. Much work has, however, focused on hospital care and physician practices with less attention on nursing home care, interdisciplinary team practices, or ongoing care of persons with chronic conditions living at home.

*Interdisciplinary Intervention Teams*

Comprehensive geriatric assessment is increasingly being used to determine an older individual's medical, psychosocial, functional, and environmental resources and problems. That assessment leads to the development of an overall plan for treatment and follow-up, which can utilize an interdisciplinary intervention team of practitioners and providers. Such practices have been shown to reduce the disability and institutionalization of older individuals. However, the effectiveness of this intervention has also been shown to vary by setting— whether, for example, it is conducted on an inpatient versus outpatient basis and by target group (i.e., it is less useful with older populations generally than it is with specific groups of older patients who have multiple or complicated conditions or who have a sudden decline or threats to the stability of their health and living situation). This is important because the time and costs involved with assessment and use of intervention teams can be significant.

## Examples of Needed Research

- Document and analyze variations in practice patterns and interventions involving older people.
- Evaluate the effect that various settings—office, hospital, nursing facility, home—have on practice patterns and treatment interventions and how health outcomes are influenced.
- Examine barriers in recognizing and treating common geriatric syndromes and their effects on outcomes.
- Explore methods to help improve practitioners' ability to discuss important and emotionally laden issues such as advance care planning (e.g., the appropriate use of simulated patients).
- Identify best care practices and their cost-effectiveness within and across various settings and for various patients.
- Test various methods to promote the use of clinical practice guidelines and other, perhaps more forceful, approaches for changing practice patterns and use of certain interventions.
- Further explore the use of advanced care planning, including how practitioners' attitudes influence its use. Suggest ways to ensure its use across numerous settings of care.

## INVOLVEMENT IN CARE DECISIONMAKING

*Methods of enhancing older individuals' and their families' involve-ment in decisionmaking about their care and its relationship to health outcomes should be explored.*

### Rationale

• Technically excellent care will not produce optimal functional health status and satisfaction if individuals are not actively engaged in managing their care.

• Older individuals' beliefs, values, and informed preferences should be an essential part of a negotiated process of treatment decisionmaking.

### Background

Increasingly, older individuals and their families are becoming actively involved in making decisions about their care and expressing their treatment preferences. Such involvement is generally seen as a much needed improvement in providing health care to older individuals, particularly with respect to decisions about care at the end of life. It is also important in achieving cooperation between professionals and patients in ongoing therapy for chronic conditions. The committee hopes that this trend of greater involvement will continue but also cautions that the basic assumption that this involvement both is wanted by older individuals and leads to better health outcomes must be investigated.

Not all people choose the same options. Individuals' feeling of autonomy, desire for independence, and willingness to accept risk affect the decisions they make and, ultimately, influence their health outcomes. Generational or cultural differences may also help explain and predict preferences. Preferences can change over time. For example, cancer patients in their 60s may be more likely to want aggressive treatment than 90-year-old patients, but such differences in preferences cannot be unilaterally assumed. Decisionmaking styles also vary, and this can have important implications for an individual's health outcomes. Kaplan and colleagues (1996) found, for example, that patients who are more passive may be at risk for poorer health outcomes than patients who are more self-reliant. Finally, preferences and goals of treatment are also likely to change if the individual develops a terminal illness.

Therefore, understanding an individual's lifestyle, expectations, preferences, and decisionmaking style is vital. This understanding can be useful not only in assessing whether an older individual's desired health outcomes were achieved but also for identifying those patients who would benefit from increased intervention.

Few individuals make decisions entirely on their own. The role of families and other concerned parties in the decisionmaking process is also important to understand. If an individual is cognitively impaired, the role played by proxy, or surrogate, decisionmakers is even more important. Proxies can provide an important perspective on the desired health outcomes of older patients. Indeed, in some instances, proxies are the only available source of information about the individual's probable decision.

However, there is little guidance available about several aspects of involving proxies in the decisionmaking process. For example, how should a proxy or proxies be chosen? This is especially difficult when more than one is available (e.g., several adult children) and they have differing views of the individual's preferences. When using proxy responses for outcomes measurement, should any special calibrations or adjustments be made to give them weights different from that of the actual individual's response? The methodology for making such adjustments with any kind of validity or reliability is very underdeveloped.

Practitioners play an important role in helping patients make choices among different treatment options. Practitioners need to be able to communicate with patients objectively, noncoercively, and sensitively and to let them know what the various outcomes are likely to be for them as individuals. Usually with older people this involves having an understanding of multivariate risk analysis or how multiple and competing risks might interact with each other. Better information on the likelihood of various events and their likely outcomes may assist effective decisionmaking, sometimes through the use of formal decision aids such as decision trees.

### Examples of Needed Research

• Include questions about expectations and values in national surveys, such as the National Health Interview Survey, Medicare Current Beneficiary Survey, and the National Nursing Home Survey to establish national norms for comparative use.

• Improve models that portray treatment benefits while taking into account competing risks and the likelihood of various events occurring.

• Establish methods of measuring patient preferences for various functional outcomes and examine how those preferences might change over time.

• Advance the use of methods that incorporate individuals' beliefs, values, preferences, and expectations into treatment plans and decisions.

• Develop methodologies for calibrating or adjusting proxy responses in outcomes measurement.

## EDUCATION AND DISSEMINATION OF OUTCOMES INFORMATION

*The effectiveness and impact on health outcomes of providing health care information to older individuals and health care professionals should be evaluated. New and improved ways of disseminating outcomes information should be tested.*

### Rationale

• Older individuals will increasingly need to make decisions about their health care.

• Outcomes information regarding the risks and benefits of their options can help them make a better informed decision.

• Outcomes information needs to be presented to older people in a form that is accessible and understandable. A variety of strategies for disseminating information exist or are being developed. Which ones will actually increase the likelihood that information will affect behavior and improve health outcomes is unknown.

### Background

More than ever before, today's older individuals face a bewildering number of choices regarding their health care. This includes not just determining which course of treatment to pursue but which health plan to join, long-term-care insurance to buy, or home health agency to employ. A variety of resources are available to help older individuals learn more about these choices. Older individuals and their families are increasingly using the Internet, interactive compact discs, and educational videos to receive health information, in addition to subscribing to more traditional health newsletters or receiving the increasing numbers of health-related publications—pamphlets, brochures, books, handouts—addressed to the public.

These educational resources also allow practically anyone to utilize the results of health outcomes research—from an older woman with breast cancer "surfing" the Internet for the latest information about treatment options to a daughter looking over performance reports of nursing facilities as she decides the most appropriate one for a parent suffering from Alzheimer's disease.

The content and method of disseminating such information will obviously need refinement. Outcomes information must be in a format that older persons can understand, particularly for those who are illiterate or have literacy problems. Alternate formats should be developed for individuals with diverse ethnic and cultural backgrounds. Other aspects of information resources also warrant attention. For example, are information resources shifting to the Internet in ways that might reduce information access for those who lack the requisite resources and skills, especially those with lower incomes and less education? Are basic information resources sufficiently keyed to the problems and needs of older age groups? Conversely, do computer resources offer new opportunities for some older individuals to be more independent in obtaining information of interest to them?

Health outcomes researchers can help determine not only what types of information older people want and need to make better choices about their health care but how this information affects practitioner behavior as well as actual health outcomes. Tremendous opportunities for improvement of patient care exist by providing practitioners with health outcomes data in an understandable and usable format. Yet, as noted by Batalden and colleagues (1994), "Telling a baseball player about his batting average (or a surgeon about his coronary artery bypass graft mortality rate) is a necessary but insufficient step toward improvement."

As more and more outcomes information is released publicly in the form of report cards and performance ratings, the effect on providers and patients needs to be monitored carefully. Schneider and Epstein (1996) recently studied the influence of Pennsylvania's *Consumer Guide to Coronary Artery Bypass Graft (CABG) Surgery* on physician referral practices and access to care. They found the guide had little credibility among referring physicians and, therefore, had little influence on their referral recommendations. Disturbingly, however, they also found that physicians believe that access to care for severely ill patients who need CABG has decreased because cardiac surgeons are no longer willing to take on patients who might hurt their ratings. Another study in New York, where a similar guide was released, found that access to care among severely ill patients had been maintained (Chassin et al., 1996).

## Examples of Needed Research

- Utilize focus groups and other kinds of qualitative research to determine what types of outcomes information older people want to make health care decisions, and the best means to present outcomes information.
- Examine how personal style and involvement in decisionmaking about care affect an individual's satisfaction and functional health status. Refine the content and method of disseminating health outcomes information.
- Evaluate whether newer forms of information dissemination, such as videotapes and interactive CD ROMs, truly enhance and improve decisionmaking.
- Investigate and improve the relevance and accessibility of on-line information resources to different groups of elderly people.
- Identify technologies that offer particular promise in making more accurate and complete patient information available for older individuals in different health care settings.

## FINANCING SYSTEMS

*Research, including randomized controlled trials and quasi-experiments, should continue to examine how various provider payment methods and programs affect the health outcomes of older individuals and populations. Outcomes of special concern are access to care, health care costs, quality of care, health-related quality of life, functional health status, and satisfaction with care.*

### Rationale

• The shift from fee-for-service to per-case and capitated payment methods is intensifying, as are efforts to reduce expenditures for certain categories of services and providers.

• Different payment schemes provide different incentives to providers and consumers that affect the accessibility, amount, mix, and quality of services available and, ultimately, the health outcomes of individuals and populations.

• Concerns about the solvency of the Medicare Part A Trust Fund as well as the impact of the aging baby boom generation on federal health spending are stimulating efforts to make further, even radical, changes in Medicare and Medicaid payment and financing methods.

### Background

Until recently, most health care organizations and practitioners were paid separately for each service provided. This type of fee-for-service payment, however, creates incentives for more services to be provided than may be necessary or appropriate. As a result, in the 1980s Medicare instituted a prospective payment system to reimburse hospitals on a per-case basis related to the patient's diagnosis and certain other factors. From the beginning, the main concern with this system has been that it will lead to the underprovision of services for each case but, absent other controls, encourage an increase in the number of cases of care. Volume performance standards have been only somewhat successful in controlling this effect and have been inequitably applied across medical disciplines.

Medicare has also sought to develop capitated payment arrangements for health plans to cover a defined set of services to enrolled individuals for a designated period of time. Plans must cover all Medicare Part A and Part B services, but they then have considerable discretion in determining what other level and mix of services to provide within their capitation rate. For Medicare enrollees in risk contracts, the Health Care Financing Administration (HCFA) currently pays an average annual per capita cost (AAPCC), based on an average cost per fee-for-service beneficiary in a geographic area (with certain adjustments for age, gender, disability status, and nursing home residence), minus 5 percent. In general, plans are at risk for losses if they exceed the total capitated payment amount for all their enrollees, but they can keep any "savings" or unused amounts rather than return them to the government.

The concern is that capitated payments create strong incentives to under-provide services or to enroll healthier individuals who need fewer services. Despite considerable research and analysis, more work remains to devise and test payment methods that do not reward health plans or practitioners for seeking the well (i.e., promoting favorable selection) and undertreating the sick (i.e., avoiding adverse selection). Another concern is that disincentives in the payment system will lead to the failure to provide certain types of care. For example, geriatric assessment requires in-depth (and hence, expensive) evaluation of an individual's functional abilities, but the administration and interpretation of these evaluations are typically not reimbursable.

Several alternative capitation methods have been suggested. Some of these alternatives have been tested (but not yet demonstrated to be satisfactory), and others are as yet untried.

### Risk Adjustment

Even though they tend to have more health problems than younger people, older people vary considerably in their health status and in the economic risks they pose to capitated health plans. Risk adjustment seeks to adjust payments to plans to better reflect actual patient or participant characteristics (i.e., plans would get more money for enrolling participants with complex medical needs). How this is done and precisely which demographic and functional "adjusters" should be included in a risk adjustment model has been the subject of much debate. Part of the debate revolves around technical questions related to data availability, quality, and predictive power. Other questions focus on possible unwanted effects of recognizing, and thereby encouraging, certain factors (e.g., past utilization of services) in the payment scheme.

### Competitive Pricing

HCFA is currently exploring the use of a competitive pricing system to set its Medicare reimbursement rates. In one planned demonstration project, all health plans in a certain region will be asked to submit bids for their estimated costs of providing a standard benefit package. Because few health plans have extensive experience with serving large numbers of very old and very frail members, concerns arise about the willingness of these plans to participate and their ability to set appropriate rates. Information is also needed on the optimum mix of high- and low-risk members, as well as the mix of private and government contracts. A health plan must accurately determine these mixes in order to be competitive in terms of benefits and services. Little is known about how these issues will interact in a rate-setting context or how the quality of care, health of members, or even costs will be affected.

*Use of Outcomes Measures to Structure Incentives*

Another approach that remains relatively untested is incorporating outcomes measures into payment incentives. Those organizations and practitioners that achieve good outcomes would receive more money. The issue of how to handle providers who do not achieve good outcomes is more problematic; if their payments are reduced, it might be more difficult for them to make needed improvements. Nonetheless, risk adjustment models need further refinement before adoption and implementation of a payment system adjusted for both risk and outcomes could serve as a strong motivation for providers to achieve good outcomes.

### Examples of Needed Research

- Conduct randomized controlled trials and quasi-experiments to test the incentives and costs of different models of reimbursement and their effect on integration and coordination of services, cost-effectiveness, and health outcomes of older individuals and their families.
- Conduct policy research to determine the impact on health outcomes of adverse and favorable selection in health plans. If appropriate, develop methods to limit favorable selection or offset the consequences of adverse selection.
- Refine risk adjustment models further.
- Identify payment methods with disincentives for providing certain types of care (e.g., not appropriately reimbursing practitioners for conducting geriatric assessments) and examine the effect on patient outcomes and costs of care.

## SERVICE DELIVERY AND UTILIZATION

*As alternative forms of organizing and delivering health care for older individuals are encouraged and continue to be developed, the effect on health outcomes should receive continuing and rigorous evaluation.*

### Rationale

• The health care system is undergoing substantial restructuring and re-organization.

• Older people and their health outcomes may be particularly affected by changes in where services are provided, by whom, how often, and in what mix and intensity.

### Background

Many of the current Medicare and Medicaid reform proposals call for beneficiaries to enroll in managed care-type health plans. However, health plans have traditionally been reluctant to become involved with older individuals in part because of fears of unlimited liability for complex care and a dearth of people willing to join (Iversen et al., 1988). Nevertheless, recent evidence from the Medicare risk program indicates that such attitudes may be changing; the number of plans entering into such contracts increased from a low of 93 in 1991 to 171 by August 1995 (GAO, 1996).

More fully integrated care delivery systems offer the potential of providing new and improved services, which could, in turn, improve health outcomes—especially for people with chronic conditions. Access to care, continuity of care, and the cost-effectiveness of care may be enhanced. The extent to which reality actually meets expectations, however, requires careful study. One issue is whether, if more care is provided and organized by an array of primary care clinicians, the benefits of coordination will exceed the possible harms to older, sicker people of being treated by those with less specialized training. Another issue is whether the emphasis on health promotion and disease prevention translates into better health status for both the more healthy and the less healthy segments of the older population.

Concerns continue to be raised that some health plans are limiting or rationing care to the detriment of their members' health. For example, plans sometimes restrict the list of prescription drugs that are covered by the plan (i.e., the plan's drug formularies). A recent study reported that this can lead to decreased quality of life, higher use of health care services, and greater health care costs (Horn et al., 1996). Likewise, utilization review policies and procedures guiding decisions about what services are medically necessary may restrict access to necessary care.

Choice of providers and access to practitioners also demand close scrutiny, particularly in underserved areas. In some rural areas, health plans enroll participants but then reject local practitioners for reasons such as lack of board certification. Such limitation of choice and potentially of access may have an impact on health outcomes. On a related note, the correlation between the usual measures of practitioner qualifications, such as board certification, and health outcomes has not been clearly established. It is also not known if this relationship, if it exists at all, varies by setting (e.g., hospital versus ambulatory care setting).

The environment in which health care organizations operate can play an important role in the way services are provided. For example, early indications from one study suggest that the probability of hospitalization for nursing home patients is substantially higher in markets with more beds per 1,000 and lower hospital occupancy rates (Mor, 1996). Similarly, the use of nursing facilities, assisted living facilities, and home health services has been shown to vary enormously by region and appears to be linked to the number and availability of these services (Delfosse, 1995). Similar variation appears to be developing as some regions begin to use hospital-based "transitional care units" or nursing home-based "subacute acute care centers" to a greater extent.

The role that geography plays in determining health outcomes also requires more study. Some research has examined how factors such as distance and topographical barriers and lack of transportation affect access to care in rural or underserved urban environments, but few studies have examined the effect such factors have on health outcomes. New telecommunication technologies offer the opportunity to increase access to care for residents in these areas, but, again, little research has been done to determine if this increased access translates into improved health outcomes.

Finally, patterns of enrollment and disenrollment may highlight some of the effects of changes in the financing and service delivery systems on older individuals' health outcomes. Some argue that greater choice in selecting health plans and practitioners will allow older individuals to "vote with their feet"; if they are dissatisfied they can simply choose another plan or practitioner. This assumption needs to be evaluated carefully by determining who disenrolls, what their medical and functional characteristics are, and where they go after disenrolling. Given Medicare's relatively open (monthly) enrollment policies, the effect of frequent disenrollment on the health plan also needs to be monitored.

### Examples of Needed Research

• Determine under what circumstances underutilization and overutilization of services have positive or adverse health and cost consequences.

- Examine the factors that have gone into health plans' decisions to serve older populations. Similarly, examine factors that will induce older people to join managed care plans.
- Evaluate whether more fully integrated care delivery systems actually provide new and improved services and, thereby, improve health outcomes—especially for people with chronic conditions.
- Determine how older individuals' health outcomes are affected by (a) the prevalence and nature of grievance and appeals procedures in health plans, (b) the extent to which they are used by the elderly (as contrasted with younger patients, and for different subgroups of the elderly, such as those with serious chronic illness), and (c) the deliberate or inadvertent barriers to their use.
- Study whether the usual measures of practitioner qualifications (e.g., board certification) correlate with good health outcomes. Determine if this possible correlation varies by setting.
- Demonstrate whether the use of nonphysician health care providers, improved systems of transporting patients, and telecommunication technology can improve health outcomes of rural and underserved populations without significantly increasing the costs of care.

## TRANSITIONS

*The impact on health outcomes when older individuals make transitions between types of care (e.g., from active treatment to palliative care), treatment settings, and health plans should be explored.*

### Rationale

• Research often has been directed at patients in specific settings (e.g., living in nursing facilities versus dwelling in the community) and in discrete health states (e.g., an acute episode of cardiovascular disease requiring hospitalization).

• Fragmentation in the health care system means older individuals are being served in multiple settings. Older adults often experience complex health patterns, undergoing multiple stages of deterioration and improvement in their health, even during a single episode of care.

### Background

There is a misperception that as people age they move along a linear continuum of care as their status gradually and smoothly changes from that of a well, active, and independent senior living in the community to that of a completely dependent nursing home resident. In reality, very few people move along such a linear path. Often the decision to move an older individual to an institutional setting where more care can be provided is put off until the individual is very disabled and in need of the highest level of care. Likewise, the goals of treatment for disease sometimes do not change from curing a patient to caring for a terminally ill patient until the disease is quite progressed. Even when chronic conditions are present, older individuals often continue to have acute care episodes.

Traditionally, health outcomes research has relied on measures of mortality to rank quality of care. The implicit assumption is that a low mortality rate equals the best possible care. For some patients, life-sustaining treatment (i.e., treatment that reduces mortality) merely prolongs dying and suffering. With an aging population now living longer than ever before, often with multiple acute and chronic problems, the health care system must become increasingly attentive to how transitions in the goals of medical care are managed. Fundamental to both geriatric and palliative care medicine is that practitioners must learn to negotiate skillfully a transition in goals of care, going from a major emphasis on extending life to an emphasis on patient comfort, even if focusing on the latter to the exclusion of the former means a patient's life is shortened. Often, however, the timing of this transition is made too late and results in adverse outcomes (SUPPORT, 1995). At the same time, real risks exist that the timing of this transition, particularly for older individuals, will occur too soon.

The current health care delivery system remains fragmented. Although improvements are being made, the interface between the settings of acute, subacute, home, ambulatory, and long-term care is not well developed. Important information about an older individual's condition or preferences may not be communicated as the individual moves between various settings. The goals of treatment and the instruments available to measure an individual's status vary for each of these different settings. Better ways of tracking patients across settings and time are needed. Finally, improved coordination of care among a variety of practitioners and care providers is also needed.

The setting of care often plays a crucial role in an individual's health outcomes; yet the effect of making a transition from one setting to another is often not well known. For example, suppose, as is often the case, that going to a nursing home even for a relatively short stay is perceived very negatively by a hospitalized patient. Perhaps the patient's long-term results would be better if he or she stayed in the hospital a little longer to receive rehabilitation services at a single site rather than be moved to a nursing home, and thus fragmenting care.

In addition to the transitions an older individual makes along the continuum of care, changes are also occurring among providers and practitioners. These changes raise questions about whether they may disrupt patterns of care and, ultimately, affect health outcomes of older people. Examples of such changes are many: physicians retire or become employees, begin to use nurse practitioners and case managers, or become part of an interdisciplinary team; physicians sometimes do not follow their patients' care into the nursing home; hospitals or clinics close; use of telephone triage may be implemented (which could have a particularly adverse effect on older individuals, who might have greater difficulty hearing or quickly comprehending verbal information); managed care contracts change hands; health systems, plans, and organizations merge or are acquired; senior management of health plans or organizations change. All of these changes have the potential of affecting the health outcomes of older people, both as individuals and as a population.

### Examples of Needed Research

• Support experiments and innovations in continuity of care and coordination of care.
• Support longitudinal research exploring the impact of transitions on health outcomes.
• Examine patient utilities for the timing and choice of transitions between care settings.
• Develop valid and reliable markers of health status to identify patients who may need to discuss a change in treatment goals.

## QUALITY ASSESSMENT AND IMPROVEMENT

*The performance of government regulatory agencies, private-sector accreditation organizations, and organizations' internal programs in using outcomes-based quality assessment and improvement systems should be evaluated for effectiveness in improving health outcomes for older populations.*

### Rationale

• Governments, private-sector accreditation organizations, and health care delivery organizations are increasingly using outcomes measures as a basis for assessing and improving the quality of care. Little is known about how effective these approaches are in terms of actually improving health outcomes.

• Depending on how they are structured and implemented, external and internal strategies for quality monitoring might contribute positively or negatively to improving desired health outcomes.

### Background

Quality can be assessed and improved by both external and internal programs. Traditional quality assurance programs were, in general, imposed by outside agencies and entities such as the federal government or private-sector accreditation organizations. They attempted to define at least minimum standards for quality and to enforce them through a variety of approaches. These approaches classically involved evaluation and audit functions; professional practices such as credentialing, peer review, and continuing education; and various kinds of licensure, certification, and accreditation. The primary focus of these external and internal quality programs was often on using structural and process measures to identify problems, determine their causes, and discipline poor individual performance.

This approach to quality assurance has, in recent years, been transformed into a quality improvement approach that focuses on how organizations can improve systems, processes, and outcomes in a continuous way. Programs using this approach are often described as "customer-" or "patient-centered," and many apply the principles of "total quality management" and "continuous quality improvement." These principles shift the focus on quality efforts from the identification of deficient individuals to the identification of opportunities to improve systems and processes in a way that will prevent quality problems and improve outcomes. Other principles emphasize scientifically and statistically based planning and assessment procedures, including the measurement of health outcomes and patient (i.e., customer) satisfaction; standardization of care processes; and feedback to practitioners of information on how their practices and results may differ from those of their peers or from evidence-based standards for practice.

In recent years, both external and internal quality programs have started to move beyond basic structure and process indicators of quality to identify whether desired outcomes are being achieved (IOM, 1990d). The Health Care Financing Administration, the Joint Commission on the Accreditation of Healthcare Organizations (JCAHO), several peer review organizations (PROs), the National Committee for Quality Assurance (NCQA), and the Foundation for Accountability (FACCT) have all begun major initiatives to identify, refine, collect, and use outcomes measures as a way to assess and improve the quality of health care. JCAHO is doing so for use in the accreditation of a variety of health care facilities and entities such as hospitals, long-term-care facilities, home health agencies, ambulatory care settings, behavioral health care organizations, health plans, and integrated delivery systems. NCQA and FACCT are identifying and developing measures and instruments to be used in evaluating health plans. The federal government's efforts have focused not only on services for Medicare and Medicaid but also on health care provided by the Departments of Defense and Veterans Affairs to military personnel and veterans. Much of the private-sector work has been stimulated by major employers' initiatives to reduce their health care spending, to determine what value is being received for this spending, and to manage more closely the health services their employees receive.

Although it is the committee's overall sense that current programs of quality management are moving in the right direction, improvements can continue to be made and different models tested. Researchers need to examine how the outcomes-oriented programs are actually being implemented and what the barriers to their successful implementation may be. For example, using certain kinds of health outcomes measures—or failing to adjust outcomes for severity of illness and comorbidities—may discourage health care organizations from serving the sickest patients.

### Examples of Needed Research

- Evaluate the effects of various approaches to external and internal quality assessment programs on health outcomes for older individuals.
- Determine if outcomes measures can effectively be used to supplement the current standards-based on-site surveys for accreditation and regulatory purposes. Evaluate the effect on outcomes of graduated approaches of quality assessment in which organizations that have bad outcomes receive more site visits and more technical assistance and those that achieve good outcomes are relieved of some reporting or survey requirements.
- Study approaches to quality assessment and management to determine how they take into account the relative values that older individuals place on

quality of care, avoidance of harm, costs of care, and other dimensions of health outcomes.

- Examine how different kinds of employers use outcomes measures to make decisions about which health plans are available to employees and covered retirees.

## REFERENCES

Batalden, P.B., E.C. Nelson, and J.S. Roberts. Linking Outcomes Measurement to Continual Improvement: The Serial "V" Way of Thinking About Improving Clinical Care. *Journal on Quality Improvement* 20(4):167–180, 1994.

Chassin, M.R., E.L. Hannan, and B.A. DeBuono. Benefits and Hazards of Reporting Medical Outcomes Publicly. *New England Journal of Medicine* 334:394–398, 1996.

Cleary, P.D., S. Edgman-Levitan, M. Roberts, et al. Patients Evaluate Their Hospital Care: A National Survey. *Health Affairs* Winter:254–267, 1991.

Delfosse, R. Urban and Rural Classification of the National Health Provider Inventory Providers: United States, 1991. *Advance Data.* No. 266. Hyattsville, Md.: National Center for Health Statistics, 1995.

Desbiens, N.A., A.W. Wu, S.K. Broste, et al. Pain and Satisfaction with Pain Control in Seriously Ill Hospitalized Adults—Findings from SUPPORT Critical Care Medicine, forthcoming.

GAO (General Accounting Office). Medicare HMOs: *Rapid Enrollment Growth Concentrated in Selected States.* GAO/HEHS-96-20. Washington, D.C.: GAO, 1996.

Greco P.J., and J.M. Eisenberg. Changing Physicians' Practices. *New England Journal of Medicine* 329:1271–1274, 1993.

Greenfield, S., L.M. Sullivan, K.A. Dukes, T.J. Tripp, and S.H. Kaplan. *Unadjusted Patient Satisfaction Scores Used in Physician Profiling Result in Spurious Ranking.* Boston: New England Medical Center, 1996.

Horn, S.D., P.D. Sharkey, and J. Gassaway. Intended and Unintended Consequences of HMO Cost-Containment Strategies: Results from the Managed Care Outcomes Project. *The American Journal of Managed Care* 2(3):237–247, 1996.

Iezzoni, L.I., ed. *Risk Adjustment for Measuring Health Care Outcomes.* Ann Arbor, Mich.: Health Administration Press, 1994.

IOM (Institute of Medicine). *Effectiveness Initiative: Setting Priorities for Clinical Conditons.* Washington, D.C.: National Academy Press, 1989.

IOM. *Acute Myocardial Infarction: Setting Priorities for Effectiveness Research.* P. H. Mattingly and K. N. Lohr, eds. Washington, D.C.: National Academy Press, 1990a.

IOM. *Breast Cancer: Setting Priorities for Effectiveness Research.* K.N. Lohr, ed. Washington, D.C.: National Academy Press, 1990b.

IOM. *Clinical Practice Guidelines: Directions for a New Program.* M.J. Field and K.N. Lohr, eds. Washington, D.C.: National Academy Press, 1990c.

IOM. *Hip Fracture: Setting Priorities for Effectiveness Research.* K.A. Heithoff and K.N. Lohr, eds. Washington, D.C.: National Academy Press, 1990d.

IOM. *Medicare: A Strategy for Quality Assurance.* K. Lohr, ed. Washington, D.C.: National Academy Press, 1990e.

IOM. *Disability in America: Toward a National Agenda for Prevention.* A.M. Pope and A.R. Tarlov, eds. Washington, D.C.: National Academy Press, 1991.

IOM. *Summary of Committee Views and Workshop Examining the Feasibility of an Institute of Medicine Study of Dying, Decisionmaking, and Appropriate Care.* Washington, D.C.: IOM1994.

Iversen, L.H., C.N. Oberg, and C.L. Polich. The Availability of Long-Term Care Services for Medicare Beneficiaries in Health Maintenance Organizations. *Medical Care* 26:918–925, 1988.

Kaplan, S.H., K.A. Dukes, L.M. Sullivan, T.J. Tripp, and S. Greenfield. *Is Passivity A Risk Factor for Poor Health Outcomes?* Boston: New England Medical Center, 1996.

Mor, V. Using Global and Targeted Outcomes Measures in Applied Settings. Presentation at the Institute of Medicine workshop "Evaluating Health Outcomes for Elderly People in a Changing Health Care Marketplace," Washington, D.C., June 20, 1996.

Patrick, D.L., H.E. Starks, K.C. Cain, R.F. Uhlmann, and R.A. Perlman. Measuring Preferences for Health States Worse Than Death. *Medical Decision Making* 14(1): 9–18, 1994.

Schneider, E.C., and A.E. Epstein. Influence of Cardiac-Surgery Performance Reports on Referral Practices and Access to Care. *New England Journal of Medicine* 335:251–256, 1996.

SUPPORT (The SUPPORT Principal Investigators for the SUPPORT Project). A Controlled Trial to Improve Care for Seriously Ill Hospitalized Patients: The Study to Understand Prognoses and Preferences for Outcomes and Risks of Treatments. *Journal of the American Medical Association* 274:1591–1598, 1995.

Task Force on Aging Research. *The Threshold of Discovery: Future Directions for Research on Aging. Administrative Document. Report of the Task Force on Aging Research.* Washington, D.C.: Department of Health and Human Services, April 1995.

# Recommendations:
# Research Infrastructure Needs

To improve the scope and quality of health outcomes research, several basic infrastructure and methodologic or analytic issues need to be addressed. As noted earlier, although the field of health outcomes research has seen a great deal of progress over the past few years, more work is still needed. Greater sophistication in data analysis and interpretation has given researchers, practitioners, and policymakers new insight, understanding, and ways to improve health care, but it has also raised more questions.

The sense of the committee is that significant breakthroughs on a variety of these questions are possible over the next 10 years. However, the committee has concerns about the current health outcomes research infrastructure—the actual workforce of health outcomes researchers and the methodologic and analytic tools used in research. The committee has made five recommendations aimed at strengthening that infrastructure. They relate to:

- **Workforce Issues**
- **Conduct of Research**
- **Data Quality**
- **Data Management Systems**
- **Methodological and Analytic Issues**

## WORKFORCE ISSUES

*Government agencies and private foundations should support training and education opportunities in health outcomes research.*

### Rationale

•   The successful implementation of an outcomes research agenda depends not only on the persuasive identification of important issues and the securing of funding but also on the availability of well-trained and committed researchers.

•   Although the private sector will provide some support, governmental and foundation aid is needed to ensure that the health outcomes research workforce is adequate in terms of overall size, appropriateness of training, and sensitivity to issues involving older individuals.

### Background

The health outcomes research workforce has two distinct components. It includes:

1. investigators and researchers who originate, design, supervise, and report basic and applied research; and
2. individuals who analyze health outcomes information and apply certain tools of health outcomes research in management, policy, and service delivery settings.

A recent IOM committee (IOM, 1995) concluded that well-trained health services researchers with practical experience in health care organizations (e.g., integrated health care systems, insurance companies) and in managing research units appear to be in short supply. A survey of employers of health services researchers, commissioned as part of that study, found that employers stated that they have the greatest difficulty in recruiting researchers with expertise in the area of "outcomes/health status measurement." Employers also indicated that within the next five years they expected to recruit more researchers in this area than in any other. However, although employers and private health plans do cover some of the costs and arrange or provide some of the care for older individuals, their primary focus is on younger age groups. Even taken as a whole, these efforts by private organizations are unlikely to substitute for more than a portion of government- and foundation-supported research and training in magnitude, coherence, scope, or concern for long-term consequences.

The Agency for Health Care Policy and Research provides some support of education and training through dissertation grants and National Research Service Awards. Other government agencies, including some components of the

National Institutes of Health, the Bureau of Health Professions, the Department of Defense, and the Department of Veterans Affairs, support varying amounts of research training that may include some attention to outcomes research. Some foundations, including the Pew Charitable Trusts and the Robert Wood Johnson Foundation, have supported education in health policy and outcomes research. More often, support from these sources comes indirectly through grants for research at academic institutions that hire investigators in training to assist in the research and learn skills on the job. Formal training support from private industry is sometimes available. For example, some private organizations sponsor students on semester or year-long internships to expose them to how health outcomes research is carried out in the for-profit environment. However, such training has typically been given to students in specific areas, such as pharmacoeconomics.

Because of their experience, expertise, and leadership positions, research training support for clinicians, especially geriatricians, will be useful in advancing the field of health outcomes research for older people. Including training in outcomes assessment as an integral part of practitioners' (physicians, nurses, dentists, etc.) initial and continuing education will also be beneficial.

## Examples of Support Needed

- Fellowships, pre- and postdoctoral traineeships, dissertation grants, grants to institutions offering health outcomes research training, loans, and other financial supports for aspiring health outcomes researchers and educational institutions.
- Health outcomes research training programs for health care professionals, especially geriatricians.

## CONDUCT OF RESEARCH

*Principles for the appropriate conduct of health outcomes research and the use and dissemination of outcomes data need to be developed and implemented.*

### Rationale

• All researchers must hold themselves to a high ethical standard of quality and integrity to maintain public confidence in the validity and integrity of their work.

• Efforts are needed to ensure that the results of health outcomes research are made available to the broader scientific community and the population at large.

### Background

The committee believes the field of health outcomes research would benefit from a statement of "principles" regarding the conduct of research. As is true in many other fields of research, concerns about the validity of the research and integrity of the researcher are bound to arise. The relationship between industry funders and independent researchers is a particular concern because of fears that industry sponsors might censor negative research results that could damage their business interests. A similar call for a professional code of ethics was issued at the 1996 annual conference of the Association for Pharmacoeconomics and Outcomes Research (Medical Outcomes and Guidelines Alert, 1996).

Ethical codes have been developed by some research organizations (e.g., the RAND Corporation and the Mayo Clinic) and other research professions. Epidemiologists, for example, have a code spelling out the researcher's obligations to the subjects of research, society, funders and employers, and colleagues. Issues covered include the need to protect the welfare of research subjects, obtain informed consent, and maintain confidential information. More generally, researchers should avoid conflicts of interest and partiality to potential sponsors, promote scrutiny of their work by describing their methods and reporting their results fully enough to limit misinterpretation, report results regardless of whether they are favorable to the sponsor's interests, take care that they choose methods appropriate to the research question, protect privileged information, and refrain from premature publication of findings. These obligations and principles should be clearly specified to funders and employers.

Resolving ethical issues will not be easy, even with the proposed code. For example, researchers at the Mayo Clinic conducted a retrospective study through the use of chart review to examine the outcomes and complication rates of silicone breast implants. They found no complications associated with the implants. Shortly after the study findings were released, attorneys for breast implant patients asked that the charts be made public so they could contest individual cases. The request has been turned down. The example highlights the conflicting demands placed on researchers. The study provided the public and other professional colleagues with important epidemiologic data on an issue with significant health and monetary implications. However, the researchers and their institution also had to protect patient confidentiality and limit the institution's liability.

## Example of Support Needed

A "statement of principles" that governs the conduct of health outcomes researchers needs to be developed and widely disseminated to health outcomes researchers and to sponsors and users of such research.

## DATA QUALITY

*Research on the quality of data used in health outcomes research should be supported.*

### Rationale

• Policymakers, consumers, managers, and others need confidence in the soundness of health outcomes information and analyses.

• Data quality varies enormously depending on the source and collection method used.

• These variations threaten the validity, reliability, and comparability of outcomes research. An understanding of data limitations and measurement problems can help users of research interpret findings with due regard for their limitations.

### Background

Although the quality of health outcomes research data is important regardless of its uses, the increasing use of outcomes data to compare health care institutions, practitioners, health plans, and services has focused much more attention on the quality of these data and the deficiencies in outcomes comparisons. Particular shortcomings relate to the sufficiency of the clinical measures of patient characteristics (including severity of illness and other risk factors), the accuracy of recording and coding patient and other data, poor identification of older persons living in rural and underserved urban areas, and the representativeness of the patient population. Because older individuals are underrepresented in some databases, attention to the generalizability of findings is also important.

Similarly, the increased interest in patient satisfaction measures as indicators of quality has prompted concerns about the improper use of well-validated measurement instruments and the use of internally developed instruments whose reliability and validity have not been tested. This threat may be particularly acute for studies undertaken and publicized by the entity that is being evaluated, especially when methods and findings are selectively reported. This has been an issue in some nursing facilities that tout internal surveys indicating high rates of satisfaction among their residents for marketing purposes, even when they also have been found to have serious and life-threatening deficiencies by state regulators.

The use of large administrative databases is very attractive for researchers because of its convenience (e.g., no primary data collection is needed); but growing concern about their limitations (e.g., the level of clinical detail available) is, on the one hand, directing health outcomes researchers to other data sources (in particular, new kinds of clinical trials) and, on the other hand, encouraging greater efforts to improve the accuracy and completeness of administrative databases and to develop techniques to compensate for their deficiencies.

## Example of Needed Research

Identify and categorize problems with the reliability, validity, and availability of data used in health outcomes research for older individuals.

## DATA MANAGEMENT SYSTEMS

*An independent appraisal of systems for data management that support outcomes research should be conducted. This includes evaluations of specific tools and applications, informatics, databases, and basic telecommunications infrastructure.*

### Rationale

• Many different systems for data management that support outcomes research have been developed.

• Each of these systems has advantages and disadvantages. Some of these systems are very expensive. Users need objective information on which to base their purchasing decisions.

### Background

The emergence of computerized data and information systems has begun to revolutionize the way health outcomes research is conducted and its results disseminated. Advanced technological applications and tools along with powerful computer software and hardware offer the possibility of conducting health outcomes research that is extremely sophisticated. For example, computerized patient records allow for gathering and utilizing more and better self-reported health-related quality-of-life information on social, economic, and spiritual issues. This type of data can then be used routinely or selectively in clinical care to monitor individual outcomes as well as in large-scale epidemiological studies. Large, data-intensive, population-based studies of health outcomes can now be conducted with newly developed technologies for collecting, linking, modeling, and analyzing data.

Researchers and users alike are confronted with a seeming overabundance of technology to assist them. Some of this technology is being very heavily marketed. Yet very little work has examined—in an unbiased manner—the advantages and disadvantages of these different technologies. The committee recommends that a *Consumers Report*-type evaluation of these various systems for data management be performed that would compare and contrast their different features. Individual purchasers could then make a more informed and objective decision about the features and products they most desire.

## Example of Needed Research

Perform independent appraisals of systems for data management to support health outcomes research. This includes evaluations of:

1. specific tools and applications (e.g., voice recognition systems, bar codes, laser wands, reminder technology);
2. informatics, databases; and
3. basic telecommunications infrastructure.

## METHODOLOGICAL AND ANALYTIC ISSUES

*Continued support should be provided to develop advances in the methodology and analysis used in health outcomes research.*

### Rationale

• Although significant progress has been made in developing new types of measurements and in improving techniques of analyzing and reporting health outcomes, much more work remains.

• With the exception of governmental support, this type of research has traditionally been difficult to fund.

• Without continued development of research methods and techniques of outcomes assessment that are in the public domain, the field of health outcomes research will be substantially impaired.

### Background

Most of the issues related to methodology and analysis have been mentioned earlier in this report. However, the committee believes it is important to highlight some of the most needed and complex methodological and analytic issues in a separate recommendation. To date, the Agency for Health Care Policy and Research (AHCPR) has been one of the most active supporters of such methodological and analytic advances. The committee is concerned that, because of recent and threatened cuts to AHCPR, this type of research will be even more difficult to fund.

### Examples of Needed Research

• Develop ways to integrate data elements across settings and over time.

• Improve methods of risk adjustment and severity measurement. These measures need to take into account patient, social, and system characteristics; they may also need to account for past treatment and patient history.

• Develop better statistical models for controlling for selection bias.

• Compare the advantages and disadvantages of different study designs (e.g., retrospective, prospective, randomized, staged qualitative).

• Determine how different scales or measures should be calibrated to increase their comparability.

• Compare the advantages and disadvantages of different approaches to gathering outcomes information (e.g., patient self-report, computer-assisted interview, chart review, review of administrative data, use of proxy information, observation of nonverbal clues, ethnographic observation). Increase the comparability of data using different approaches.

• Expand techniques to obtain information from people who are cognitively impaired.

- Determine when outcomes should be measured. Establish a standard definition of an "episode" of care. Examine how time of measurement affects the outcome result (e.g., measuring satisfaction each time services are provided and averaging them versus measuring it once a year).
- Develop better statistical models for determining selection bias.
- Study how measures of utility and patients' preferences relate to summary measures of health-related quality of life.

## REFERENCES

IOM (Institute of Medicine). *Health Services Research: Workforce and Educational Issues.* M.J. Field, R.E. Tranquada, and J.C. Feasley, eds. Washington, D.C.: National Academy Press, 1995.

*Medical Outcomes and Guidelines Alert.* At First APOR Meeting, Challenges and Controversies. 4(10):6–8, 1996.

# APPENDIX
# Workshop Agenda and Participants

*Evaluating Health Outcomes for Elderly People in a*
*Changing Health Care Marketplace*

June 20, 1996
Institute of Medicine
Washington, D.C.

## WORKSHOP AGENDA

**8:00**   Welcoming remarks and overview of workshop agenda
John Eisenberg, Committee Chair

**8:15**   **Users:** The Questions We Want Health Outcomes Research to Answer

Moderator: Paul Schyve, Joint Commission on Accreditation of Health-care Organizations
Consumers: Ann Wyatt, National Citizens' Coalition for Nursing Home Reform
Mary Jo Gibson, American Association of Retired Persons
Practitioners: Steven Levenson, Genesis Healthcare
Plan Providers: Sandra Harmon-Weiss, U.S. HealthCare Systems
Nursing Home Provider: Jan Olson, Wilder Foundation Residence West
Congress: Charles Kahn, III, House Ways and Means Health Sub-committee
HCFA: Stephen Jencks, Health Care Financing Administration

**10:00**  **Markets:** How the Health Care Market Affects Elderly People's Health Outcomes

Presenter: William Weissert, University of Michigan
Discussant: Peter Fox, PDF Consulting

**10:45**  **Individuals:** Measuring Satisfaction and Other Patient Perceptions

Presenter: Joan Teno, The George Washington University
Discussant: Susan Edgman-Levitan, Picker Institute

**11:30–12:30 Organizations:** Using Global and Targeted Outcomes Measures in Applied Settings

Presenter: Vincent Mor, Brown University
Discussant: Richard Besdine, Health Care Financing Administration

**1:30–4:00 Participants' Research Recommendations**

Participants were asked to present their recommendations to the committee regarding the types of health outcomes research for elderly people they would like to see undertaken in the next 10 years. The following topics were suggested as a guide, but recommendations on other topics were also welcome:

Market and Organizational Issues
(e.g., market structure/incentives, quality improvement, interpreting and disclosing outcomes research)

Individual Characteristics
(e.g., frail elderly, terminally ill patients, diversity, dementia, patient preferences)

The Conduct of Health Outcomes Research
(e.g., measurement of quality of life, severity adjustment)

**4:30   Workshop ends**

## WORKSHOP PARTICIPANTS

Elena M. Andresen
Associate Professor
Department of Community Health
Saint Louis University School of
  Public Health
St. Louis, MO

Linda Hiddemen Bardondess
Executive Vice President
The American Geriatrics Society
New York, NY

Richard Besdine
Director
Health Standards and Quality Bureau
Health Care Financing Administration
Baltimore, MD

Barbara Chapman
U.S. General Accounting Office
Washington, DC

Carolyn Clancy
Acting Director
Center for Outcomes and Effectiveness
  Research
Agency for Health Care Policy and
  Research
Rockville, MD

Mary Ellen Courtright
FHP Foundation
Long Beach, CA

Teresa A. Dolan
Acting Associate Dean
University of Florida College of Dentistry
Gainesville, FL

Molla S. Donaldson
Division of Health Care Services
Institute of Medicine
Washington, DC

Joyce Dubow
Public Policy Institute
American Association of Retired Persons
Washington, DC

Susan Edgman-Levitan
Executive Director
Picker Institute
Boston, MA

John M. Eisenberg
Chairman and Physician-in-Chief
Department of Medicine
Georgetown University Medical Center
Washington, DC

Lynn Etheredge
Consultant
Chevy Chase, MD

Charles J. Fahey
Marie Ward Doty Professor of Aging
  Studies
Fordham University
Bronx, NY

Judith Feder
Professor of Public Policy
Institute for Health Care Research and
  Policy
Georgetown University
Washington, DC

Peter Fox
PDF Consulting, Inc.
Chevy Chase, MD

Mary Jo Gibson
Director, Health Policy Research
American Association of Retired Persons
Washington, DC

Dorothy Gordon
The Johns Hopkins University School of
  Nursing
Baltimore, MD

Sandra Harmon-Weiss
Vice President and Medical Director
U.S. Healthcare
Blue Bell, PA

Jennie Harvell
Program Analyst
Office of the Assistant Secretary for
  Planning and Evaluation
Department of Health and Human Services
Washington, DC

Dick Hegner
Senior Research Associate
National Health Policy Forum
Washington, DC

Roger Herdman
Senior Scholar
Institute of Medicine
Washington, DC

Alene Hokenstad
Director, Home Care Innovation Project
United Hospital Fund
New York, NY

Anne Jackson
Professor of Nursing, Emerita
City University of New York
Sarasota, FL

Stephen F. Jencks
Senior Clinical Advisor
Health Standards and Quality Bureau
Health Care Financing Administration
Baltimore, MD

Charles N. Kahn, III
Staff Director, Health Subcommittee
Committee on Ways and Means
U.S. House of Representatives
Washington, DC

Rosamond Katz
Assistant Director, NGB-Health Finance
U.S. General Accounting Office
Washington, DC

Don Keller
U.S. General Accounting Office
Washington, DC

Pamela Kerin
AARP Andrus Foundation
Washington, DC

Janet Kline
Congressional Research Service
Washington, DC

Marianne Laouri
Director, Quality Improvement and
    Outcomes Research
PacifiCare Health Systems
Cypress, CA

Barbara Lardy
Director
Health Promotion and Disease Prevention
American Association of Health Plans
Washington, DC

Steven Levenson
Physician Services Division
Genesis Healthcare
Baltimore, MD

Robert McCartney
Denver, CO

Peggy McNamara
Association for Health Services Research
Washington, DC

Vincent Mor
Director, Center for Gerontology and
    Health Care Research
Brown University
Providence, RI

Evvie Munley
American Association of Homes and
    Services for the Aged
Washington, DC

Thomas Obiesesan
Chief, Section of Geriatrics
Department of Medicine
Howard University Hospital
Washington, DC

Jan Olson
Director of Nursing
Wilder Foundation Residence West
Saint Paul, MN

Marcia Ory
National Institute on Aging
Bethesda, MD

Anu Pemmarazu
Committee on National Statistics
National Research Council
Washington, DC

Eleanor M. Perfetto
Director, Health Outcomes Assessment
Wyeth-Ayerst Research
Philadelphia, PA

Daniel Perry
Executive Director
Alliance for Aging Research
Washington, DC

Susan Pettey
American Medical Directors Association
Columbia, MD

Liliana Pezzin
Agency for Health Care Policy and
  Research
Rockville, MD

Linda J. Redford
Director, National Resource and Policy
  Center on Rural Long Term Care
Center on Aging
University of Kansas Medical Center
Kansas City, KS

Alan Rosenbloom
American Association of Homes and
  Services for the Aged
Washington, DC

Lisa Rubenstein
Associate Clinical Professor of Geriatric
  Medicine
University of California, Los Angeles
Acting Chief, Ambulatory Care and
  General Internal Medicine
Veterans Administration Medical Center
Sepulveda, CA

Judith Salerno
Department of Veterans Affairs
Washington, DC

Joanne Schwartzberg
Director, Department of Geriatric Health
American Medical Association
Chicago, IL

Paul M. Schyve
Senior Vice President
Joint Commission on Accreditation of
  Healthcare Organizations
Oakbrook Terrace, IL

Sushil Sharma
Program Evaluation and Methodology
  Division
General Accounting Office
Washington, DC

Cathy D. Sherbourne
Behavioral Scientist
Social Policy Department
The RAND Corporation
Santa Monica, CA

Brenda Spillman
Researcher
Agency for Health Care Policy and
  Research
Rockville, MD

Robyn Stone
Deputy Assistant Secretary
Office of Disability, Aging, and Long
  Term Care Policy
Department of Health and Human Services
Washington, DC

Eric G. Tangalos
Associate Professor of Medicine
Mayo Medical School
Section Head, Geriatric Medicine
Division of Community Internal Medicine
Mayo Clinic
Rochester, MN

Joan Teno
Associate Director
Center to Improve Care of the Dying
The George Washington University
Washington, DC

Jürgen Unützer
Assistant Professor
Department of Psychiatry
University of Washington School of
  Medicine
Seattle, WA

Joan F. Van Nostrand
Statistician
National Center for Health Statistics
Hyattsville, MD

Anne Voss
Manager, Outcomes Research
Ross Product Division
Abbott Laboratories
Columbus, OH

Andrew Webber
Consumer Coalition for Quality
  Health Care
Washington, DC

William G. Weissert
Professor, Health Policy and
  Administration
School of Public Health
Research Scientist
Institute of Gerontology
University of Michigan
Ann Arbor, MI

Nancy Whitelaw
Associate Director
Center for Health System Studies
Henry Ford Health System
Detroit, MI

Mark E. Williams
Director, Program on Aging
University of North Carolina School of
  Medicine
Chapel Hill, NC

Alicia Wilson
Health Outcomes Assessment
Wyeth-Ayerst Research
Philadelphia, PA

Ann Wyatt
Home Care Associates Institute, and
Board Member, National Citizens'
  Coalition for Nursing Home Reform
Bronx, NY

# Bibliography

The reference works listed here are additional sources drawn upon by the committee. The works are arranged according to their relevance to particular recommendations made in the report.

## HEALTH-RELATED QUALITY OF LIFE

Cassel, C.K. Issues of Age and Chronic Care: Another Argument for Health Reform. *Journal of the American Geriatrics Society* 40:404–409, 1992.

Gill, T.M., and A.R. Feinstein. A Critical Appraisal of the Quality of Quality-of-Life Measurements. *Journal of the American Medical Association* 272(8):619–626, 1994.

Gurwitz, J.H., N.F. Col, and J. Avorn. The Exclusion of the Elderly and Women From Clinical Trials in Acute Myocardial Infarction. *Journal of the American Medical Association* 268:417–1422, 1992.

Lawrence, R.H., and A.M. Jette. Disentangling the Disablement Process. *Journal of Gerontology: Social Sciences* 51(B):4, S173–S182, 1996.

Patrick, D.L., and P. Erickson. *Health Status and Health Policy: Allocating Resources to Health Care.* New York: Oxford University Press, 1993.

Rubenstein, L.V., D.R. Calkins, S. Greenfield, et al. Health Status Assessment for Elderly Patients: Report of the Society of General Internal Medicine Task Force on Health Assessment. *Journal of the American Geriatrics Society* 37:562–569, 1988.

Spilker, B., F.R. Molinek, K.A. Johnston, et al. Quality of Life Bibliography and Indexes. *Medical Care* 28(12):DS1–DS77, 1990.

Stewart, A.L., C.D. Sherbourne, and M. Brod. Measuring Health-Related Quality of Life in Older and Demented Populations. In *Quality of Life and Pharmacoeconomics in Clinical Trials*, 2d ed. B. Spilker, ed. Philadelphia: Lippincott-Raven Publishers, 1996.

Testa, M.A., and D.C. Simonson. Assessment of Quality-of-Life Outcomes. *New England Journal of Medicine* 334:(13)835–840, 1996.

## SATISFACTION WITH CARE

Gertis, M., S. Edgman-Levitan, J. Daly, and T.L. Delbanco. *Through the Patient's Eyes: Understanding and Promoting Patient-Centered Care.* San Francisco: Jossey-Bass, Inc., 1993.

Owens, D.L., and C. Batchelor. Patient Satisfaction and the Elderly. *Social Science and Medicine* 42(11):1483–1491.

Rothman, M.L., P. Diehr, S.C. Hedrick, W.W. Erdly, D.G. Nickinovich. Effects of Contract Adult Day Health Care on Health Outcomes and Satisfaction with Care. *Medical Care* SS75–SS83, 1993.

Teno, J. Consumer Reports and Ratings of Medical Care: Will We Ever Get Satisfaction? Paper presented at the Institute of Medicine workshop "Evaluating Health Outcomes for Elderly People in a Changing Health Care Marketplace," Washington, D.C., June 20, 1996.

## "TOOLBOX" OF OUTCOMES MEASURES AND A CORE SET OF OUTCOMES MEASURES

Andresen, E.M., B.M. Rothenberg, and J.G. Zimmer, eds. *Health Status Assessment Among Older Adults.* New York: Springer Publishing Co., in press.

Magaziner, J. The Use of Proxy Respondents in Health Studies of the Aged. In *The Epidemiologic Study of the Elderly.* R.B. Wallace and R.F. Woolson, eds. New York: Oxford University Press, 1992.

Mor, V. Using Global and Targeted Outcomes Measures in Applied Settings. Presentation at the Institute of Medicine workshop "Evaluating Health Outcomes for Elderly People in a Changing Health Care Marketplace," Washington, D.C., June 20, 1996.

Stewart, A.L., and J.E. Ware, eds. *Measuring Functioning and Well-being. The Medical Outcomes Study Approach.* Durham, N.C.: Duke University Press, 1992.

## PRACTICE PATTERNS AND THEIR EFFECT ON OUTCOMES

### General

Chassin, M., J. Kosecoff, R. Park, et al. Does Inappropriate Use Explain Geographic Variations in the Use of Health Care Services? A Study of Three Procedures. *Journal of the American Medical Association* 258:2533–2537, 1987.

Wennberg, J.E., and M.M. Cooper. *Dartmouth Atlas of Health Care in the United States.* Chicago: American Hospital Association, 1996.

Wennberg, J.E., and A. Gittelsohn. Small Area Variations in Health Care Delivery: A Population-Based Health Information System Can Guide Planning and Regulatory Decisionmaking. *Science* 182:1102–1108, 1973.

Wennberg, J.E., J.L. Freeman, R.M. Shelton, and T.A. Bubolz. Hospital Use and Mortality Among Medicare Beneficiaries in Boston and New Haven. *New England Journal of Medicine* 321(17):1168–1173, 1989.

### Advance Care Planning

Emanuel, L.L., and E.J. Emanuel. Decisions at the End of Life: Guided by Communities of Patients. *Hastings Center Report* 23(5):6–14, 1993.

The SUPPORT Principal Investigators for the SUPPORT Project. A Controlled Trial to Improve Care for Seriously Ill Hospitalized Patients: The Study to Understand Prognoses and Preferences for Outcomes and Risks of Treatments. *Journal of the American Medical Association* 274:1591–1598, 1995.

Thomasma, D.C. The Ethical Challenge of Providing Healthcare for the Elderly. *Cambridge Quarterly of Healthcare Ethics* 4(2):148–162, 1995.

### Clinical Practice Guidelines, Pathways, and Other Strategies

Berwick, D.M. Harvesting Knowledge from Improvement. *Journal of the American Medical Association* 275(11):877–878, 1996.

Epstein, R.S., and L.M. Sherwood. From Outcomes Research to Disease Management: A Guide for the Perplexed. *Annals of Internal Medicine* 124(9):832–837.

Greco P.J., and J.M. Eisenberg. Changing Physicians' Practices. *New England Journal of Medicine* 329:1271–1274, 1993.

Institute of Medicine (IOM). *Clinical Practice Guidelines: Directions for a New Program.* M.J. Field and K.N. Lohr, eds. Washington, D.C.: National Academy Press, 1989.

IOM. *Guidelines for Clinical Practice: From Development to Use.* M.J. Field and K.N. Lohr, eds. Washington, D.C.: National Academy Press, 1992.

### Interdisciplinary Intervention Teams

Applegate, W.B., and R. Burns. Geriatric Medicine. *Journal of the American Medical Association* 275(23):1812–1813, 1996.

Rubenstein, L.Z., D. Wieland, and R. Bernabei. *Geriatric Assessment Technology: The State of the Art.* Milan, Italy: Editrice Kurtis, 1995.

Stuck, A.E., A.L. Siu, G.D. Wieland, J. Adams, and L.Z. Rubenstein. Comprehensive Geriatric Assessment: A Meta-Analysis of Controlled Trials. *Lancet* 342:1032–1036, 1993.

## INVOLVEMENT IN CARE DECISIONMAKING

Flood, A.B., J.E. Wennberg, R.F. Nease, F.J. Fowler, J. Ding, and L.M. Hynes. The Importance of Patient Preferences in the Decision to Screen for Prostate Cancer. *Journal of General Internal Medicine* 11(6)342–349, 1996.

Fryback, P.D., and B.R. Reinert. Facilitating Health in People with Terminal Diagnoses by Encouraging a Sense of Control. *Medsurg Nursing* 3(2):197–201, 1993.

Kaplan, S.H., K.A. Dukes, L.M. Sullivan, T.J. Tripp, and S. Greenfield. *Is Passivity A Risk Factor for Poor Health Outcomes?* Boston: New England Medical Center, 1996.

Welch, G.H., P.C. Albertsen, R.F. Nease, T.A. Bubolz, and J.H. Wasson. Estimating Treatment Benefits for the Elderly: The Effect of Competing Risks. *Annals of Internal Medicine* 124(6):577–584, 1996.

## EDUCATION AND DISSEMINATION OF OUTCOMES INFORMATION

Batalden, P.B., E.C. Nelson, and J.S. Roberts. Linking Outcomes Measurement to Continual Improvement: The Serial "V" Way of Thinking About Improving Clinical Care. *Journal on Quality Improvement* 20(4):167–180, 1994.

Chassin, M.R., E.L. Hannan, and B.A. DeBuono. Benefits and Hazards of Reporting Medical Outcomes Publicly. *New England Journal of Medicine* 334:394–398, 1996.

Schneider, E.C., and A.E. Epstein. Influence of Cardiac-Surgery Performance Reports on Referral Practices and Access to Care. *New England Journal of Medicine* 335:251–256, 1996.

## FINANCING SYSTEMS

Physician Payment Review Commission (PPRC). *Annual Report to Congress.* Washington, D.C.: PPRC, 1996.

Weissert, W. Outcomes Research in Managed Care for Elderly People: A Review and Agenda. Paper presented at the Institute of Medicine workshop "Evaluating Health Outcomes for Elderly People in a Changing Health Care Marketplace," Washington, D.C., June 20, 1996.

## SERVICE DELIVERY AND UTILIZATION

Delfosse, R. Urban and Rural Classification of the National Health Provider Inventory Providers: United States, 1991. *Advance Data.* No. 266. Hyattsville, Md.: National Center for Health Statistics, 1995.

GAO (General Accounting Office). *Medicare HMOs: Rapid Enrollment Growth Concentrated in Selected States.* GAO/HEHS-96-20. Washington, D.C.: GAO, 1996.

Horn, S.D., P.D. Sharkey, and J. Gassaway. Intended and Unintended Consequences of HMO Cost-Containment Strategies: Results from the Managed Care Outcomes Project. *The American Journal of Managed Care* 2(3):237–247, 1996.

Iezzoni, L.I., ed. *Risk Adjustment for Measuring Health Care Outcomes.* Ann Arbor, Mich.: Health Administration Press, 1994.

Iversen, L.H., C.N. Oberg, and C.L. Polich. The Availability of Long-Term Care Services for Medicare Beneficiaries in Health Maintenance Organizations. *Medical Care* 26:918–925, 1988.

Mor, V. Using Global and Targeted Outcomes Measures in Applied Settings. Presentation at the Institute of Medicine workshop "Evaluating Health Outcomes for Elderly People in a Changing Health Care Marketplace," Washington, D.C., June 20, 1996.

## TRANSITIONS

Bauer, E.J. Transitions from Home to Nursing Home in a Capitated Long-Term Care Program: The Role of Individual Support Systems. *Health Services Research* 31(3):309–326, 1996.

Coleman, B., E. Kassner, and J. Pack. *New Directions for State Long-Term Care Systems. Vol. II, Addressing Institutional Bias and Fragmentation.* Washington, D.C.: American Association of Retired Persons/Public Policy Institute, 1996.

Newman, S.J. *The Effects of Supports on Sustaining Older Disabled Persons in the Community.* Washington, D.C.: American Association of Retired Persons/Public Policy Institute, 1995.

## QUALITY ASSESSMENT AND IMPROVEMENT

IOM. *Medicare: A Strategy for Quality Assurance.* K.N. Lohr, ed. Washington, D.C.: National Academy Press, 1990.

Kane, R.L. Improving the Quality of Long-Term Care. *Journal of the American Medical Association* 273(17):1376–1380, 1995.

## CONDUCT OF RESEARCH

Angell, M. *Science on Trial: The Clash of Medical Evidence and the Law in the Breast Implant Case.* New York: W.W. Norton, 1996.

Beauchamp, T., R. Cook, W. Fayerweather, G. Raabe, S. Cowles, and G. Spivey. Ethical Guidelines for Epidemiologists. *Journal of Clinical Epidemiology* 44(Suppl. 1):151S–169S, 1991.

Hillman, A.L., J.M. Eisenberg, M.V. Pauly, B.S. Bloom, H. Glick, B. Kinosian, and J.S. Schwartz. Avoiding Bias in the Conduct and Reporting of Cost-Effectiveness Research Sponsored by Pharmaceutical Companies. *New England Journal of Medicine* 324(19):1362–1365, 1991.

## DATA QUALITY

Harris, T.B., and M.G. Kovar. Data Sets for Research in Aging: The National Center for Health Statistics. In *The Epidemiologic Study of the Elderly.* R.B. Wallace and R.F. Woolson, eds. New York: Oxford University Press, 1992.

Committee on National Statistics. *Priorities for Data on the Aging Population: Summary of a Workshop.* Washington, D.C.: National Academy Press, 1996.

IOM. *Health Data in the Information Age: Use, Disclosure, and Privacy.* M.S. Donaldson and K.N. Lohr, eds. Washington, D.C.: National Academy Press, 1994.

Schneider, R.E., P. Martus, and A. Klingbeil. Reversal of Left Ventricular Hypertrophy in Essential Hypertension. A Meta-Analysis of Randomized Double-Blind Studies. *Journal of the American Medical Association* 275(19):1507–1513, 1996.

Schulz, K.F, I. Chalmers, D.A. Grimes, et al. Assessing the Quality of Randomization from Reports of Controlled Trials Published in Obstetrics and Gynecology Journals. *Journal of the American Medical Association* 272(2):125–128, 1994.

U.S. Congress, Office of Technology Assessment. *Identifying Health Technologies That Work: Searching for Evidence.* OTA-H-608. Washington, D.C.: U.S. Government Printing Office, 1994.

## METHODOLOGICAL AND ANALYTIC ISSUES

Fowler, F.J., P.D. Cleary, J. Magaziner, et al. Methodological Issues in Measuring Patient-Reported Outcomes: The Agenda of the Work Group on Outcomes Assessment. *Medical Care* 32(7 Suppl.):JS65– JS76, 1994.

Parker, S.G., X. Du, M.J. Bardsley, et. al. Measuring Outcomes in Care of the Elderly. *Journal of the Royal College of Physicians of London* 28(5):428–433, 1994.

Sullivan, L.M., K.A. Dukes, L.H. Harris, et al. A Comparison of Various Methods of Collecting Self-Reported Health Outcomes Data Among Low-Income and Minority Patients. *Medical Care* 33(4 Suppl.):AS183–AS193, 1995.

Weinberger, M., B. Nagel, J.T. Hanlon, et al. Assessing Health-Related Quality of Life in Elderly Outpatients: Telephone Versus Face-to-Face Administration. *Journal of the American Geriatrics Society* 42(12):1295–1299, 1994.